Monographien aus dem Gesamtgebiete der Psychiatrie

20

Psychiatry Series

Herausgegeben von
H. Hippius, München · W. Janzarik, Heidelberg
C. Müller, Prilly-Lausanne

Richard M. Torack

The Pathologic Physiology of Dementia

*With Indications for Diagnosis
and Treatment*

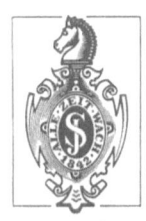

Springer-Verlag
Berlin Heidelberg New York 1978

Professor Dr. RICHARD M. TORACK, Washington University, School of Medicine, Department of Pathology, 660 South Euclid Avenue, St. Louis, MO 63110/USA

ISBN-13: 978-3-642-88439-9   e-ISBN-13: 978-3-642-88437-5

DOI: 10.1007/978-3-642-88437-5

Library of Congress Cataloging in Publication Data. Torack, Richard M., 1927 –. The pathologic physiology of dementia, with indications for diagnosis and treatment. (Monographien aus dem Gesamtgebiete der Psychiatrie; v. 20). Bibliography: p. Includes index. 1. Dementia. I. Title. II. Series. RC386.2.T67. 616.8'9. 78-15102.

2123/3130-543210

Contents

1. Historical Overview of Dementia

The evolution of senile dementia has traditionally been considered to represent an aspect of senescence which, in turn, is the normal final phase of human performance that occurs as a prelude to death. Yet there has always been vast disagreement regarding the meaning of this statement. Let us begin with senescence itself (Tibbitts, 1957):

> The character of elderly men – men who are past their prime may be said to be formed for the most part of elements that are the contrary of all those in youth. They have lived many years; they have often been taken in, and often made mistakes; and life on the whole is a bad business. (Aristotle, 384–322 B.C.).

Aristotle's negataive opinion is exactly opposite that of his mentor Plato as he presents his plan for gerontocracy (Tibbitts, 1957):

> And he who at every age, as boy and youth and in mature life, has come out of the trial victorious and pure, shall be appointed a ruler and guardian of the State; he shall be honored in life and death.
> There can be no doubt that the elder must rule to younger. (Plato, 427–347 B.C.).

A very astute appraisal of aging was that of Cicero in his famous essay "De Senectute" (Couch, 1959):

> The blame seems to me misdirected. If the faults are due to old age, the same misfortunes would have befallen me and other men, but I have known many men who have no complaints. (Cicero, 106–43 B.C.).

The controversy regarding aging inevitably transfer to that condition we call senile dementia, since as senility, it personifies the ultimate force of aging. There have always been those who advocate the concept that senility, like senescence, is that bad product of brain aging and decay to which all of us will succumb if we live long enough. Their adversaries argue that this idea is untenable because there is no age by which everyone has been shown to become senile. The complexity of this problem is evidenced by the fact that this issue has not been resolved despite the efforts of modern medical science. The history of dementia affords an opportunity to understand how the present situation evolved. There is another benefit that accrues from a study of history, one which was described very well by Harry Truman in his memoirs (Truman, 1956):

> I learned of the unique problems of Andrew Johnson, whose destiny it was to be thrust suddenly into the presidency to fill the shoes of one of history's great leaders. When the same thing happened to me, I knew just how Johnson had coped with his problems, and I did not make the mistakes he made.

Prelude to the Modern Era

One initial impact of mental problems like dementia was the result of the fact that changes in the brain accompanied the disorder. This indicated a relationship between mind and brain, which certainly was appreciated by Hippocrates, who discussed the nature of consciousness in his book, *Sacred Disease* (Jones, 1923):

> Wherefore I assert that the brain is the interpreter of consciousness. Some people say that the heart is the organ with which we think, and that it feels pain and anxiety. But is not so . . . Men ought to know that from the brain, and from the brain only, arise our pleasures, joys, laughter and jests, as well as our sorrows, pains, griefs and tears. Through it, in particular, we think, see, hear, and distinguish the ugly from the beautiful, the bad from the good, the pleasant from the unpleasant . . . It is the same thing which makes us mad or delirious, inspires us with dread and fear, whether by night or by day, brings sleeplessness, inopportune mistakes, aimless anxieties, absentmindedness, and acts that are contrary to habit. These things that we suffer all come from the brain, when it is not healthy.

Hippocrates seems to be concerned with the notion that the heart, rather than the brain, is the organ of the mind, so we can assume that many people believed this to be true. His concept of mind and brain was perpetuated by Galen, who not only affirmed this view, but added a belief that dementia was due to a "coldness in the brain". However, the collapse of Rome and Greco-Roman culture ushered in an era of intellectual confusion in which the fears of Hippocrates were confirmed. The mind moved from the brain to the heart. Presumably, the nature of this heroic age required an association between consciousness, strength, and heart. At any rate, this alien habitat seems like a good explanation for the intellectual confusion. Our heritage from this era is best manifest in the rich endowment of our vocabulary linking heart with all those things that Hippocrates talked about: hearty, heartfelt, hartless, heart strings, heartache, etc. The whole idea culminates in the sentiment expressed on Valentines Day. For those who only believe the dictionary, one current definition of heart is: "the vital center of one's being, emotions and sensibilities; the seat or repository of emotions."

Hippocrates and Galen were resurrected during the renaissance along with Socrates and Plato and, at this time, the relationship between mind and brain was renewed. Although renaissance man adopted the classics, he also felt compelled to enlarge and improve this culture by his own hunger for knowledge. Among other things, brains were studied avidly and one of the points of greatest interest was the ventricular system with its fluid content. This is a direct outgrowth of the concern with body humors in the medical classics. This interest expanded when Harvey published his theory on the circulation of blood in 1628. The circulation of a fluid peculiar to the brain was considered by some to have comparable importance for mental performance. Some astonishing ideas of brain function were formulated and those of René Descartes achived greatest notoriety.

In Descartes, we find that renaissance ideal of "universality" expressed in a completeness comparable to Da Vinci. Primarily a mathematician, he produced essays on music, on the development of the fetus, and on legal doctrine. Late in life, he became obsessed with the function of the mind; his "Je pense donc je suis" is still a milestone in the history of philosophy. He was also engrossed in the topic of matter and mind (or soul). Complicating his science was a strong religious conviction, which embodied God as an infinite source, a fountainhead. He conceived of the brain as another spiritual system, needing a similar initiator of all activity. He ascribed this power to the pineal gland which has been ridiculed ever since Descartes' folly (Haldane and Ross, 1911):

It is, "the principal seat of the soul, and the place where all its thoughts occur." As the "animal spirits, which are like a tenuous wind, or rather like a pure or vital flame", pass along "the passage from the anterior to the posterior cavities of the brain", it takes advantage of its strategic position (it is "suspended above the passage") to exert itself upon them, and is reciprocally affected by the changes they undergo." (Descartes, 1596–1650.)

Within a short time, Gall and those who followed him showed that the neocortex was the seat of consciousness and any similar function of the pea-sized pineal was considered absurd. However within the past decade, we have learned that the pineal gland synthesizes powerful neurohormones and that these "animal spirits" do move through the third ventricle to affect the pituitary gland and probably vital nuclei in the hypothalamus and medulla as well. And Descartes did it all with deductive reasoning and lyric prose.

The first investigator to localize consciousness to the cortex was Joseph Gall (Ackerknecht, 1958). By 1810, he had formalized a new concept of brain function that was based mainly on 12 proofs he derived from comparative anatomy of the brain. His initial conclusions were fourfold:

1. Faculties are innate.
2. Faculties depend on organic structures.
3. The brain is the organ of all faculties, tendencies, and feelings.
4. The brain is composed of as many organs as the individual has faculties, tendencies, and feelings.

Gall observed that the development of these faculties paralleled the evolution of the neocortex, so he localized these organs in the cortex but, while his anatomy was revolutionary, his physiology was his downfall. He believed whenever a certain faculty like memory was highly developed, an appropriate part of the cortex was enlarged. This in turn led to certain protuberances of the skull. Finally he conceived that he could palpate and influence these organs through an intact skull. This was the beginning of phrenology and the ending of science.

The real impact of evolution occurred in the last half of the nineteenth century, in large measure this was inspired by Darwin. At this time the neocortex was precisely defined anatomically and Sherrington was the unquestioned leader in localizing different levels of brain function. However, his methodology was not well suited for a study of consciousness; this remained a task for Hughlings Jackson, using human disease as the experimental model. Jackson related consciousness to his highest centers, which he identified in various parts of the cortex but in which he recognizes several levels (Taylor, 1931). In epilepsy, he says:

There are three degrees of negative affection of consciousness; in clinical language they are mental confusion, insensibility and coma.

His conception of insanity was even more important for he believed this to be the result of a dissolution of the various levels of consciousness:

In every insanity, with one obvious exception (complete dementia), there is a double symptomatic condition, a condition of two opposite mental elements, one negative and one positive (or superpositive). Repeating what has just been said, there is in every insanity (1) negatively, defect of consciousness (loss of some consciousness) and there is (2) the consciousness remaining.

In complete dementia, the situation becomes quite different:

Here the negative mental affection is greatest, is indeed total; there is dementia. There are no positive symptoms; there is no mind or consciousness. There is complete dissolution, and thus no lower range of evolution remains. Here is what I called "the obvious exception" to the statement that the mental condition in insanities is a double condition, one of a negative and a positive element. In this depth there is no person but only a living creature. (Hughlings Jackson, 1834–1911.)

Following the stimulus of Jackson's ideas, insanity was recognized as brain disease and not the result of an indwelling evil spirit, or a just tribute exacted by an intemperate and dissolute life. This was an abnormality of the neocortex and the primary brain change was cortical atrophy.

During this same interval the clinical manifestations of dementia were being re-evaluated and reclassified. Prior to this time mental illness was distinguished on the basis of activity (mania, melancholia) and on the time of life (adolescence, menopause, senium, etc.). Now Maudsley (1868) and Clouston (1874) in England, Charcot (1868) in France, and Kraepelin (1883) in Germany were furiously characterizing the various forms of insanity. Probably the best example of this new psychiatry is the evolution of dementia praecox (schizophrenia), which occurred in the eight editions of Kraepelin's textbook *Psychiatrie* that appeared between 1883 and 1910.

A major advance occurred when it became clear that only certain forms of insanity were associated with cortical atrophy. These chiefly occurred after age 65 and, because this was believed to be due to brain aging, the entity was called senile dementia. Conversely most of the insanities occurring at an earlier age had no change in the brain organ. We must appreciate that although the new entities were considered to represent abnormal brain function, no one had any idea of the basis of the problem or of a rational form of treatment. Indeed the situation had been unchanged since Pinel took the chains off the mental patients in the Bicêtre in 1793.

The insanity related to degeneration of the brain was chronic, progressive, and fatal. By 1868 Maudsley was able to characterize several categories of chronic insanity:

They represent in undistinguishable varieties the shattered wrecks of the mental organization. Three main groups of them may perhaps be made. The first will consist of those who exhibit a few striking delusions which seem to be automatically expressed.

In a second group of cases there is a more general incoherence or craziness, without any particular delusion, but with greater external activity.

Lastly, there is a group of demented patients in whom the mind is almost extinguished: who have to be fed, moved, clothed, and cared for; who evince little or no sensibility; whose only utterance is a grunt, a whine, or a cry; and whose only movements are to rub their heads or hands.

These chronic progressive disorders were even less treatable than the functional problems but some idea of cause was derived from the brain changes. In 1874, Clouston could write about the cause of senile insanity on the basis of 203 cases occurring in subjects over the age of 60:

The three great dangers to normal mental senility are hereditary brain weakness, a diseased vascular system, and the effects of over exertion or toxic irritations of brain structures either at the time or at former periods of life which have left the convolutions weakened.

It is impossible to fix an age at which physiological senility begins, and therefore we cannot fix an age for senile insanity.

Premature age in look characterizes many of those who become insane after 45.

By the end of the century, sophistication but no fundamental change in Maudley's concept had occurred. Senile dementia had become a disease entity comprising two forms. Simple senile dementia appeared to be the comparatively benign form, beginning with episodes of confusion that gradually became complicated by loss of memory and increasing apathy. Within another group the memory loss was attended by emotional abnormalities, anxiety, hyperactivity, paranoia, melancholia, or depression, which could be confused with nonprogressive affective disorders. This group became the presbyophrenia of the next decade. Finally each of these could lead to a third stage in which a virtual destruction of consciousness and self were dramatically present.

Age of Alzheimer and Kraepelin

The 20 years from 1890 to 1910 probably witnessed the most dynamic events in the history of mental illness. Kraepelin reorganized the entire content of psychiatry while Alzheimer characterized the brain changes whenever they occurred. In the background was the restless giant, Sigmund Freud. During most of this time he was frustrated in his attempts to proselytize his new radical approach to mental illness but a the end, he erupted on a triumphant tour to America. The real heroes are still being debated.

Emil Kraepelin was the king of psychiatry (Kahn, 1959; Braceland, 1957). He graduated from medical school in 1878 at the University of Würzburg. Then he spent the next 4 years with Gudden in Munich, who must have impressed Kraepelin mightily, for all his books are dedicated to him. Yet he was unhappy with psychiatry. He left Munic and returned to Leipzig to study psychopharmacology. He wanted to leave psychiatry but Wundt, his new mentor, talked him into writing a handbook of psychiatric diseases, which he did largely for economic reasons. Now he was forced to confront the very issues that troubled him. While medicine, in general, was establishing firm disease entities through clinical-pathologic correlation, psychiatry was muddling along with its traditional descriptive brand of nosology. Terms like "monomania melancholia attonita (metaphysical hair splitting and bodily inaction)" could have been used just as easily by Galen. Having organized his own thoughts, he wrote a pocket-sized small book, about three-fourths of an inch thick, during the Easter recess in 1882.

This *Compendium der Psychiatrie* was published in 1883 and it was eminently successful in many ways. First of all, Kraepelin made enough money so that he could marry his childhood sweetheart, Miss Ina Schwabe, in 1884. Secondly, he was convinced that he should remain in psychiatry. Finally, he was launched on a career in which he established classes of mental disease, based upon objective analysis of course, outcome, and cause. This was done through the medium of his text book, the title of which was simplified to *Psychiatrie*. In its grand eighth edition published between 1909 and 1915, that little pocket book had evolved to four volumes and 3048 pages.

In 1891, Kraepelin returned to Germany, as Professor of Psychiatry at Heidelberg, and the next 12 years are reputed to have been the happiest of his life. He surrounded himself with some of the best minds in Europe. In his clinics and laboratories, discussions of the nature of mental illness became explorations in clinical astuteness, pathologic correlation, and speculation on etiology. This frenzy of inquiry became translated into the fourth edition of *Psychiatrie* in 1893, the fifth edition in 1896, and the sixth edition in 1899. In this way he defined and redefined concepts of dementia praecox, manic-depression, paranoia, and paraphrenia most notably, but along with the entire content of psychiatric disease.

In 1903, Kraepelin was enticed away from his storyland to Munich by the offer of a grand new clinic and laboratory, which represented the big opportunity to study the causes of the new diseases he was creating. He established a multidisciplinary method of investigation, which was to evolve into the internationally renowned *Deutsche Forschungs- anstalt für Psychiatrie*. This was the instrument that he felt was necessary to establish mental disease on a firm scientific basis. Twenty chairs were provided for pathology alone. Anatomy, physiology, and chemistry laboratories were also lavishly appointed and staffed with the best men available. His choice to head the prestigious pathology department was Alzheimer, who had come to Heidelberg in 1902. In Munich, both the new institute and the textbook *Psychiatrie* flourished. The fame of the seventh edition in 1904 established him as the leader of world psychiatry.

As Kraepelin classified psychiatric diseases, he relied chiefly on course and outcome, but as an astute nosologist, he realized that absolute distinction could be achieved only by a recognition of cause. Unfortunately, very few mental diseases had a recognized etiology, the big notable exception being syphilis. The problem was that entities, such as schizophrenia, were accompanied by no recognizable brain change, so that pathologic study was of no help. The only category, apart from syphilis, in which brain change occurred regularly was in the insanities of the aged.

About half of these people had cerebral infarcts, so that arteriosclerosis was identi- fied as the cause of dementia in this group of patients. However most of the remainder had cortical atrophy without evidence of infarction and many had no significant arterio- sclerosis. In 1899, a young neuropathologist called Alzheimer published an article in which he claimed that this noninfarct dementia was also due to vascular disease, but one which involved arterioles rather than arteries. This arteriolosclerosis could only produce a local ischemia, severe enough to kill nerve cells but not to create an infarct. This explanation apparently was not very satisfying to Kraepelin, for he discusses this prob- lem in the seventh edition of *Psychiatrie* in the following words:

> Arteriosclerotic changes in the brain are very common in the senile period of life, yet it is doubt- ful if one is justified in considering them only as evidence of early senility, particularly in view of the fact that extensive arteriosclerosis may exist without mental impairment. One must conclude either that the vascular disease in arteriosclerotic insanity is not, in spite of its great similarity, identical with that occurring in normal senility, or that in the former case the vascular change is an accompani- ment of only secondary importance in a disease process which is highly destructire of nerve tissue.

Alois Alzheimer, in many respects, is the antithesis of Kraepelin. Born in a small town in Bavaria, he nonetheless appears to have had the economic affluence to pursue his academic ideals. Throughout his career, he maintained an interest in both clinical and pathologic aspects of disease. Apparently he was a meticulous and precise worker, but not an innovator. In writing of his collaboration with Franz Nissl at Frankfurt am Main, Lewey (1970) who knew both men remarks:

> One might guess that the flood of startling ideas was Nissl's, but that it was Alzheimer who demonstrated histologically, the correctness of the premises.

Kraepelin also appears to have been more impressed with Nissl, for he called him to Heidelberg in 1895, whereas it was 1902 before Alzheimer got a similar call. At any rate, this must have evolved into a close association, because Kraepelin took Alzheimer with him to Munich the following year. The imaginative leadership of Kraepelin and the opulent appointment of the new laboratories were put at Alzheimer's disposal. In this atmosphere, Alzheimer flourished. He achieved the status of Professor Extraordinarius in 1908, but more important, he became recognized as a foremost morphologist and teacher. He left Munich to assume the chair of psychiatry at the University of Breslau in 1912. He died 3 years later from rheumatic heart disease.

Almost as soon as Kraepelin reached the pinnacle of power, he had to be concerned about maintaining his position. The real threat to Kraepelin's position of preeminence was not his failure to identify etiologic agents for his diseases, rather it was the psycho-analytical movement, which established mental illness independently of brain chemistry or structure. This is diametrically opposed to the organic theory of mental illness. The originator of this concept, Sigmund Freud, was an exact contemporary of Kraepelin, both men having been born in 1856. But in 1890, while Kraepelin is on the brink of international fame, we find Freud in an insignificant staff position at the Institute for Children's Diseases in Vienna. However, this prosaic appointment was to provide Freud with the experience he needed to organize his embryonic thoughts on psychological trauma to the subconscious mind.

The idea of a subconscious mind did not originate with Freud, rather it can be traced back to Anton Mesmer and his concept of animal magnetism. In its simplest form, Mesmer believed that forces existed in the universe that affected a level of mental performance outside the area of immediate awareness. The idea of celestial influence of human events is as old as astrology, but Mesmer added a new personal dimension by his belief that these forces created a mental conflict between two levels of consciousness. This was particularly prominent during the phase of the full moon, a phenomenon from which we derive the term lunatic. His solution to the problem was to release the turmoil by a contact with the subconscious mind. He attempted to do this by his experiments with hypnotism.

Mesmer was a very controversial figure and hypnotism did not achieve credibility until it was adopted by Charcot (Owen, 1971). One should more than muse how the "Founder of Neurology" and the master of clinical-pathologic correlation could become so involved with such an abstract concept as the subconscious mind. As the "Caesar of the Salpêtrière" he had defined Parkinsons's disease, multiple sclerosis, miliary aneu-rysms, amyotrophic lateral sclerosis, and complications of tabes dorsalis among other things. In all of these studies, he was as passionately dedicated to pathologic anatomy as he was to clinical medicine. But, as he became more involved with the neuroses, espe-cially hysteria, he realized that he was dealing with a clinical disorder with no pathologic counterpart. Unlike Kraepelin, Charcot was able to shed his organicity and, in this case, he came to the conclusion that he was dealing with an illness that was of psychic origin rather than due to a change in the brain organ.

Once Charcot had accepted a psychic origin for these disorders, he had to relate this to a level of mental performance of which the person was not aware. This is the real beginning of the subconscious mind. Next, like Mesmer, he had to devise some technique to contact or influence this second level of mental function. Charcot seems to have been introduced to hypnotism by a Dr. Azam of Bordeaux who experimented with it at least as early as 1859. Similar trials began in Paris in 1878. When Freud came to Paris in 1885, hypnotism was an established technique in the management of hysteria.

In 1885 Freud obtained a travel grant to study in Germany, but instead he went to Paris to work under Charcot. He was not very happy there and stayed less than 5 months. Nonetheless this was sufficient time for him to be very impressed with Charcot's differentiation of hysterical paralysis, his ideas about the subconscious mind and its manipulation with hypnosis. Back in Vienna, his post at the Children's Hospital afforded an excellent opportunity to observe patterns of psychic trauma during childhood. In Freud's own words, we can see how these became linked with sex activity (Riviere, 1966):

> Influenced by Charcot's view of the traumatic origin of hysteria, one was readily inclined to accept as true and as aetiologically significant the statements made by patients in which they ascribed their symptoms to passive sexual experiences in the first years of childhood – to put it bluntly to seduction.
> This reflection was soon followed by the discovery that fantasies are created to cover up the auto erotic activity of the first years of childhood, to embellish it and raise it to a higher plane. And now, from behind the fantasies the whole range of a child's sexual life came to light. (Freud, 1856–1939).

Freud continued to expand these ideas and by 1895 he had formulated a theory of parental seduction as a cause of mental disease. These findings, which he presented in a series of three lectures on the etiology of hysteria to the Doctor Kollegium in Vienna, were quite well received by the general practioners in attendance. This encouraged him to speak on the same subject to the prestigious Society of Psychiatry and Neurology in May of the following year. Kraft-Ebing was the chairman of this elite group and, when Freud finished, he disdainfully remarked, "This sounds like a scientific fairy tale". Freud was crushed and he never again addressed the Society.

Regardless of his critics and detractors, Freud was offering something that they could not do and that was quite remarkable. He was proposing a cause and, even more important, a cure for mental illness. He substituted psychoanalysis and interpretation of dreams for hypnosis as the technique by which repressed psychological trauma could be identified and raised to the level of consciousness. When this was achieved, the abnormal behavior was to be resolved.

The emphasis on sexual trauma offended sensibilities and the denial of brain change outraged the establishment. There was only one aspect of psychoanalysis that was admirable – it worked. A major breakthrough occurred in 1902, when Bleuler, a well-respected psychiatrist, agreed to try the technique in his clinic in Switzerland. Five years later, there was another milestone: A.A. Brill came to Bleuler's clinic.

A.A. Brill was a young psychiatrist from America who was on the verge of despair because of his inability to treat mental patients. He went to Bleuler's clinic and learned about psychoanalysis. When the returned to New York, he was an ardent convert, the St. Paul of the new Psychiatry. Brill was a very effective champion and psychoanalysis spread remarkably in America. In 1909, Freud and Jung were invited to speak at Clark University in Worcester, Mass., to give a series of lectures on psychoanalysis before a very sophisticated audience. The series of five lectures was received with considerable applause, especially by James Putnam, the Professor of Neuropathology at Harvard. After this reception, it was just a matter of time before a new king of psychiatry would be crowned.

Needless to say, Freudian psychiatry was totally unacceptable to Kraepelin, who was seeking a brain change, morphologic or chemical, as the explanation for mental illness. But the hostility and ridicule of the organists obviously was not working very well. The situation was intensified when Bleuler broke ranks and agreed to test psychoanalysis. Bianchi condemned psychoanalysis in his textbook of 1905, but by then, it was obvious that only some new indicator of brain change in dementia could solve the dilemma. And the chief burden of discovering such a marker fell on the grand institute of Kraepelin's in Munich. After all, that was the primary reason for its existence.

The magic marker, which was to dispel this frustration temporarily, was remarkably slow in its evolution. In 1889, Ramon y Cajal and his metallic impregnation techniques demonstrating glial histology were accorded recognition by the German Anatomical Society at the University of Berlin. Blocq and Marinesco (1892) had modified these methods so that they were able to show a new structure, destined to become known as the senile plaque, in a brain from an elderly epileptic. There is no mention of dementia at this time. These bodies were not described again until Redlich (1898) noted them in two cases of senility and atrophy, probably because one of these patients also had epilepsy. Even then, another 6 years were to elapse before Alzheimer (1904) reported their presence in other cases of senile dementia. One must wonder why Alzheimer did not get more excited about the senile plaques. First of all, the metallic stains he used at that time were not supposed to stain neural structures, so he assumed that they were glial in origin. Secondly, he still believed that the basic problem was arteriolosclerosis, and senile plaques had an infrequent relationship to any vascular structure.

The most urgent need was for a new technique to evaluate neurons. Nissl's basophilic stains had revealed acute and chronic neuronal abnormalities but no convincing changes were ever seen in mental disease. The breakthrough occurred in 1903 when Max Bielschowsky completed his own studies on metallic impregnation and showed that he could stain threadlike structures in neurons, which he called neurofibrils. We do not know when Alzheimer learned how to do this, but in 1906, he used the technique to study the brain of a 55-year-old female with a 4.5-year history of progressive dementia. He saw numerous senile plaques but in addition, he saw something entirely new. The neurons contained a marked thickening of neurofibrils, which Alzheimer called neurofibrillary tangles. At last here was tangible proof of neuronal disease. Alzheimer presented his discovery as a case report at a meeting of the South West German Society of Alienists in Tübingen. The report covers little more than one page and has no recorded discussion (Wilkins and Brody, 1969).

Alzheimer was certain that this was a new disease entity:

In summary, we are apparently confronted with a distinctive disease process. An increasing number of unusual diseases have been discovered during the past few years. These observations show that we should not be satisfied to take a clinically unclear case and by making great efforts, fit it into one of the known disease categories.

A distinction between early- and late-onset dementia was not established before Alzheimer although this seems to be a very plausible idea. These cases of early onset were comparatively rare and the dementia was not very different from the more common late-onset group, but there is a natural reluctance to believe that dementia at 50 is the same as dementia at 75, especially if the latter is due to aging. This seems to be one reason why the distinction made by Alzheimer was so widely accepted. Within the next 5 years another 11 cases appeared in the literature including one more by Alzheimer himself (Table 1.1). Several of these already referred to this problem as "Alzheimers's disease". A closer look at the events of these years seems to be advisable.

The first clinicopathologic evaluation of these new cases was published by Perusini (1909). This report consisted of four cases including Alzheimer's original case and a subsequent case published by Bonfiglio in 1908. Perusini was obviously in close contact with Alzheimer. Not only was Alzheimer's case included with his description of neurofibrillary tangles, but he also mentioned the case of a 31-year-old syphilitic with senile plaques, who was studied by Alzheimer. Apparently, both men agreed that these cases

Table 1.1 Summary of cases of Alzheimer's disease reported 1907–1911

Author	Sex	Age at death (years)	Age at onset (years)	Dura-tion (years)	Memory loss	Stage I Spatial dis-orientation	Apathy	Stage II Agnosia	Apraxia	Aphasia	Stage III Seizures	Severe dementia	Pathology NF[a]	SP[b]
Alzheimer (1907)	F	55	51	4.5	+	+		+		+		+	+	+
Bonfiglio (1908)	M	68	63	5	+	+			+			+	+	+
Sarteschi (1909)	F	69	64	5	+		+	+				+	+	+
Perusini (1909)	M	46	37	9	+	+			+	+	+	+	+	+
Perusini (1909)	F	65	62	3	+		+			+		+	+	+
Barrett (1910)	M	68	50	18	+	+		+	+	+		+	+	+
Alzheimer (1911)	M	59	56	3	+	+	+	+	+	+	+	+	+	+
Bielschowsky (1911)	F	60	58	2	+		+	+	+	+		+	+	+
Lafora (1911)	M	61	56	5	+	+	+			+		+	+	+
Fuller (1911)	M	56	54	2	+	+	+		+	+		+	+	+
Betts (1911)	F	62	55	7	+	+			+	+	+	+	+	+
Schnitzler (1911)	F	36	31	4	+		+					+	+	+
Jansens (1911)	F	58	53	5	+				+	+	+	+	+	+

[a] NF, neurofibrillary tangles.
[b] SP, senile plaques.

were sufficiently unique to merit distinction, primarily from Fischer's cases of presbyo-phrenia, in which 19 of 37 had tangles as well as plaques.

Now we must return to Kraepelin, who was preparing his eighth edition of *Psychia-trie.* Available to him were the cases reported by Perusini and probably another case, reported by Sarteschi in 1909. Alzheimer appears to have convinced him of the distinc-tion from senile dementia, but only just. In the book, his description comes at the very end of his chapter on the aging brain and it is presented quite equivocably ...

> The clinical significance of Alzheimer's disease is at present still unclear. While the anatomic find-ings suggest that this condition deals with an especially severe form of senile dementia, some circum-stances speak to a certain extent against this, namely the fact that the disease may arise even at the end of the 5th decade. One would describe such cases at least in terms of "Senium Praecox", if not more preferably that this disease is more or less independent of age.

His remarks conclude with a recognition of variable apraxia, agnosia, and aphasia, which tend to offer distinction from presbyophrenia. In effect Kraepelin is saying that the pathology may be characterized by quantitative but not qualitative differences from senile dementia, that the presence of aphasia, agnosia, and apraxia can distinguish this from senile dementia, but they are not always present, and in consequence, the best argument for distinction is the age of onset.

This then was the great endorsement, appearing in the second volume of the eighth edition published in 1910, that is usually cited as the reason Alzheimer's disease became established. There is no doubt that despite all the qualifying remarks, Alzheimer's disease was accepted as a distinct entity immediately. In 1911, Bierschowsky, Fuller, Jansens, and Lafora referred to "Alzheimer's disease" in their descriptions of presenile dementia. The recognition is even more amazing if one looks at the major clinical and pathologic features of the 13 cases recorded within the 5-year interval ending in 1911 (Table 1.1). Memory loss and terminal severe dementia occurred in all, but these findings were also characteristic of senile dementia. Age of onset varied between 31 and 64, with 5 cases occurring outside the previously prescribed age limit of 40–60. Two cases did not mani-fest any evidence of localized cortical dysfunction, agnosia, apraxia, and aphasia, and only 3 included all of these defects. Seizures were present in only 4 cases. One case did not have plaques. Neurofibrillyry tangles were found in every case; however, they are also found in late-onset dementia.

Bielschowsky's stain was a great success and pathologists the world over used it to study every form of mental disease. By the end of 1912, more than 45 articles appeared in the literature reporting the occurrence of senile plaques and neurofibrillary tangles in all forms of dementing disease. Since this material comprised at least 500 brains, certain conclusions appeared justified:

1. Plaques and tangles do not appear in dementia paralytica (syphilis).
2. They are not characteristic of affective disorders (even though a manic-depressive aged 79 had senile plaques).
3. They can be found in arterisclerosis with multiple focal softenings, but usually in small numbers, which are considered insufficient to explain the dementia. Most inves-tigators believe that they occur independently of vascular disease.
4. The most comspicuous occurrence of both changes is in presenile dementia.
5. Senile plaques and a variable number of neurofibrillary tangles are present in senile dementia.
6. Normal senium can be associated with these changes but they are present in small numbers.

This means that by 1912, any concerned individual knew all those facts about plaques and tangles that were used, 30 years later, to discredit the specificity of these changes. So the real question is why these findings were not considered to be important in 1912. The answer seems to involve the intellectual and emotional attitudes of that era, which were not present in the next generation. The reputation of Alzheimer as an accomplished neuropathologist and even the halfhearted endorsement by the authority, Kraepelin, were certainly important. The new morphology, revealed by silver impragnation, added a new dimension to the study of the brain. This type of cellular change was not found in any other organ and, quite naturally, it would be expected to be associated with distinctive brain dysfunction. But the real impact occurred in the ideologic struggle, which is personified by Kraepelin and Freud. The organic psychiatrists welcomed these neuronal changes with open arms, because they refuted the idea that sex was more important than brain matter in the causation of mental illness. Alzheimer's disease was even more important to neuropathlogists because, if Freud was right, they could lose their jobs. In reality, neither Alzheimer nor Kraepelin established Alzheimer's disease; it was Freud, who did so.

History of Alzheimer's Disease

The controversy that was present at the beginning of the establishment of Alzheimer's disease as an entity has continued to the present time. Curiously the argument never involved Alzheimer himself. He was the major beneficiary of the early success of the new morphology. The acceptance of presenile dementia as a distinct entity and the fame this brought with it led to his appointment as Chairman of Psychiatry at the University of Breslau in 1912. Unfortunately little achievement remained for him. He developed rheumatic heart disease and died in 1915. More than 50 years later a Ciba Symposium on "Alzheimer's Disease and Related Diseases" convened in London. W.H. McMenemey paid this salute to Alzheimer:

> It is fitting that, in our tribute to the memory of Alzheimer, we should feel it necessary to review both the clinical and pathological aspects of the disease, and I would ask those, who decry the use of eponymic terms in medicine, what alternative name workers in the second decade of this century could have used?

For the others, Emil Kraepelin and Sigmund Freud, neurofibrillary tangles and senile plaques were to have little consequence. The main issue that divided them concerned those mental problems in which these brain changes did not occur.

Emil Kraepelin did not complete his "magnum opus" until 1915. By this time, World War I was in full fury and European medicine was more concerned with gunshot wounds than psychotic behavior. In the meantime, the psychoanalytical movement was sweeping across America. Eventually Freud would even have the temerity to publish his scathing psychoanalysis of the most prominent American of that age, Woodrow Wilson. Actually there was little that Kraepelin could do to diminish the rising impact of psychoanalysis. He was a master of clinical analysis and classification, but he could not derive an effective form of treatment from these brilliant discourses. After the contribution of Alzheimer, no new insight into the nature of mental disorder emanated from the grand institute in Munich. A ninth edition of *Psychiatrie* appeared in 1927, 1 year after his death, but

Kraepelin only edited volume 2. Volume 1 was taken over by Lange and volumes 3 and 4 were reproduced from the eighth edition.

His fame continued to diminish under the influence of time and the success of psychoanalysis. This brillaint classifier of mental disease was mentioned in *Founders of Neurology* only in relation to assistants and students. The psychiatry of Freud was dominant until tranquilizers proved to be more effective than psychoanalysis in the treatment of functional mental disease. The effectiveness of these drugs stimulated the research that has led to the currently popular chemical basis of these disorders. The present status of neurochemistry in psychiatric research and therapy is a remarkable epitaph to Kraepelin but, like so many other visionaries, he was a man before his time.

Senile plaques and neurofibrillary tangles had little meaning for Freud. Any onset of a mental problem de novo after 50 and especially after 65 years of age could hardly be related to parental seduction. If he considered any link with sex life, he probably concluded that this was a fitting end to these aged who had lost their sex appetite.

However, this overview really concerns the distinction of presenile dementia from senile dementia and ultimately the relationship of both the normal aging. Kraepelin had considered the age of onset as a most distinguishing characteristic but the neuropathologists, who were proselytizing this disorder, regarded the morphologic changes to be of equal significance. In this way, the presence of plaques and especially of neurofibrillary tangles in a young person with dementia became Alzheimer's disease. That is why both Lafora's and Schnitzler's cases were so diagnosed even without any focal clinical syndrome. This diagnostic specificity of senile plaques and neurofibrillary tangles was the earliest of the three criteria to fall into disrepute. We have noted earlier that senile plaques were known to occur, not only in nondemented old patients, but also in cases of brain disease, such as epilepsy and syphilis unaccompanied by dementia, even prior to the eighth edition of *Psychiatrie*. Neuropathologists seem to have regarded tangles as being more important than plaques, despite the fact that 10 of Fisher's 37 cases of presbyophrenia had tangles as well as plaques. Schnitzler's case was called Alzheimer's disease without plaques, but there is no case in the literature without tangles. The subsequent recognition of tangles in Parkinson's disease, in amyotrophic lateral sclerosis and, more sporadically, in a wide variety of chronic degenerative brain diseases effectively destroyed any concept of specificity. In order to rescue the diminishing stature of pathology, Grunthal (1930) suggested that granulovacuolar changes in neurons had greater specificity for Alzheimer's disease than either tangles or plaques. These peculiar cytoplasmic changes had been described by Simchowitz in 1910 and they had been noted regularly since that time. This prop was not very effective, for within 6 years, Jervis and Soltz (1936) were to argue for the clinical distinction of Alzheimer's disease as the specific aspect of the disease.

When senile plaques and neurofibrillary tangles lost their significance, the concept of exaggerated or premature aging suffered proportionately. This in turn led to a revival of a vascular basis for these dementias, which was really quite similar to that proposed by Alzheimer before he discovered tangles. Curiously the stimulation of this theory was not provided by a neuropathologist or even a psychiatrist, rather it was the effort of a famous gastroenterologist Walter Alvarez. Alvarez was interested in the nervous system but mainly as it affected the stomach. It was the emotional trauma of watching his brilliant father-in-law, a college president, deteriorate with dementia in his fifties, that made Alvarez consider the basis of this decline. Like so many before him, he could not believe that aging had any etiologic significance for a person of this age. Instead he proposed that small-artery disease was causing local cerebral ischemia to produce small strokes. The cumulative effect of such damage was mental decay. That is what Alzheimer said in 1899.

During this era of clinical predominance, the basis for distinction between senile dementia and Alzheimer's disease was early onset plus the presence of agnosia, aphasia, and apraxia. These *Herdsymptome* were believed to indicate a different involvement of the neocortex than that found in dementia over 65. Once again Kraepelin was correct for it was only a matter of time until the specificity of these findings was also disproven. Acutally Sourander and Sjögren (1970) attempted to prove the specificity of the diagnostic triad and they wound up doing exactly the opposite. In 68 cases of Alzheimer's disease diagnosed on these clinical criteria, they found that age of onset was between 45 and 59 in 50%, between 60 and 64 in 30%, and between 65 and 69 in 20%. Only two conclusions were possible. Either the progress of medicine in the last 70 years had succeeded in delaying the onset of senility from 60 to 70 years of age or there was no dementing syndrome that was dinstinctive for presenile dementia. Today, the latter choice is believed to be correct.

Our last consideration is the diagnosis of Alzheimer's disease that is based upon age. It is important to remember that aging is a clinical entity and not a pathologic category of diesease. Medical problems that occur in the elderly are the same as those that are present in the young. For this reason they are considered to be age-related and not due to age itself. For example, old people die of cancer and heart disease that is identical to these conditions occurring in persons under 65. This is why Alzheimer initially considered senile dementia to be vascular disease rather than aging. But senile plaques changed this entire approach because they were not associated with the vasculature and because they were found in the nondemented elderly. This seemed to be a pathologic correlate to the clinical concept of mental aging, typified by forgetfulness and mental confusion. The presence of similar complaints early in dementia is the basis of every consideration of this disorder as exaggerated aging.

The intriguing paradox of this situation is that age now assumes the stature both of a chronologic event and an etiologic agent. Every nosologist appreciates the hazardous aspect of this ideology. This pitfall is realized when the same conditions occurs in middle age, rather than in senescence. Now there is an interaction of concept that proceeds as follows: If aging is a disease process, by definition it cannot occur in the young. Therefore, an abnormality that occurs in the young must be distinct from aging. That is precisely what Kraepelin intimated and what Alvarez publicized. After 70 years we have come to the realization that there is no basis for either a clinical or pathologic distinction of adult dementia before or after the age of 65. Now we must attempt to decide whether the entire process is aging itself or some age-related disorder. Then we can decide on a new name.

References

Ackerknecht, E.R. (1958): Contributions of Gall and the phrenologists to knowledge of brain function. In: The Brain and its Function. Wellcome Historical Medical Library. Oxford: Blackwell, pp. 149–153

Alvarez, W.C. (1946): Cerebral arteriosclerosis with small commonly unrecognized apoplexies. Geriatrics 1, 159–166

Alzheimer, A. (1899): Beitrag zur pathologischen Anatomie der Seelenstörungen des Greisenalters. Neurol. Centralbl. 18, 95–96

Alzheimer, A. (1904): Histologische Studien zur Differenzialdiagnose der progressiven Paralyse. Nissls Arbeiten 1, 18

Alzheimer, A. (1907): Über eine eigenartige Erkrankung der Hirnrinde. All. Z. Psychiatr. 64, 146–148

Alzheimer, A. (1911): Über eigenartige Krankheitsfälle des späteren Alters. Z. Neurol. Psychiatr. 4, 356–385

Barrett, A.M. (1910): Degeneration of intracellular nuerofibrils with miliary gliosis in psychoses of the senile period. Proc. Am. Med. psychol. Assoc. 17, 303

Betts, J.B. (1911): On the occurrence of nodular necroses (Drüsen) in the cerebral cortex. A report of twenty positive cases. Am. J. Insan. 67, 43–56

Bielschowsky, M. (1903): Die Ziele bei Impregnation der Neurofibrillen. Neurol. Centralbl. 22, 997–1006

Bielschowsky, M. (1911): Zur Kenntnis der Alzheimerschen Krankheit (präsenilen Demenz mit Herdsymptomen). J. Psychol. Neurol. 18, 273

Blocq, P., Marinesco, G. (1892): Sur les lésions et la pathogenie de l'épilepsie dite essentielle. Semin. Med. 12, 445–446

Bonfiglio, F. (1908): Die speciali reperti in un caso di probabile sifilide cerebrale. Rivista sperim. freniatria 34, 196

Braceland, F.J. (1957): Kraepelin, his system and his influence. Am. J. Psychiatry 114, 871–876

Charcot, J.M. (1881): Clinical Lecture on Senile and Chronic diesease. London: New Sydenham Soc.

Clouston, T.S. (1884): Clinical Lectures on Mental Disease. Philadelphia: Leas and Son, pp. 628–655

Couch, H.N. (1959): Cicero on the Art of Growing Old. Ilfracombe: A.H. Stockwell

Fischer, O. (1907): Miliare Nekrosen mit drüsigen Wucherungen der Neurofibrillen usw. Monatsschr. Psychiatr. Neurol. 22, 361

Fischer, O. (1910): Die presbyophrene Demenz, deren anatomische Grundlagen und klinische Abgrenzung. Z. Neurol. Psychiatr. 3, 371–471

Fuller, S.C. (1911): A study of the miliary plaques in brains of the aged. Proc. Am. Psychol. Assoc.

Fuller, S.C. (1912): Alzheimer's disease (senium praecox): The report of a case and review of published cases. J. Nerv. Ment. Dis. 39, 440–455, 536–557

Grünthal, E. (1930): Alzheimersche Krankheit. In: Bumke's Handbuch der Geisteskrankheiten. Berlin: Springer, Vol. II

Haldane, E.S., Ross, G.R.T. (Translat.) (1911): The Philosophical Works of Descartes. Cambridge: University Press, pp. 345–347

Jansens, G. (1911): Ein Fall der Alzheimerschen Krankheit. Cas. Beitr. Psychiatr. Neurol. Bladen 4, 5

Jervis, G.A., Soltz, S.W. (1936): Alzheimer's disease – the so-called juvenile type. Am. J. Psychiatr. 93, 39–56

Jones, W.H.S. (Transl.) (1923): Hippocrates: The Sacred Disease in Select Works. London: Heinemann, Vol. 2, pp. 139–183

Kahn, E. (1959): The Emil Kraepelin memorial lecture. In: Epidemiology of Mental Disorder. Pasamanick, B. (ed.). Am. Assoc. Adv. Sci. 60, 1–38

Kraepelin, E. (1883): Compendium der Psychiatrie. Leipzig: Barth

Kraepelin, E. (1910): Psychiatrie, 8th Edition. Leipzig: Barth, Vol. 2, pp. 616–632

Kraepelin, E. (1912): Psychiatrie, 7th Edition. Abstracted by A.R. Diefendorf. London: MacMillan, pp. 333–341

Lafora, G.R. (1911): Beitrag zur Kenntnis der Alzheimerschen Krankheit oder präsenilen Demenz mit Herdsymptomen. Z. Ges. Neurol. Psychiatr. 6, 15–20

Lewey, F.J. (1970): Alois Alzheimer. In: The Founders of Neurology. W. Haymaker (ed.). Springfield: C.C. Thomas, pp. 165–168

16

Maudsley, H. (1868): The Physiology and Pathology of Mind. London: MacMillan, pp. 404–411

McMenemey, W.H. (1970): Alois Alzheimer and his diesease. In: Alzheimer's Disease and Related Conditions. Wolstenholme, G.E.W., O'Connor, M. (eds.). London: Churchill, pp. 5–9

Owen, A.R.C. (1971): Hysteria, Hypnosis and Healing. The Work of J.M. Charcot. London: Dobson

Perusini, G. (1909): Über klinisch und histologisch eigenartige psychische Erkrankungen des höheren Lebensalters. Nissl-Alzheimers Arbeiten 3, 297

Redlich, E. (1898): Über miliare Sklerose der Hirnrinde bei seniler Atrophie. Jahrb. Psychiatr. Neurol. 17, 208–216

Riviere, J. (Transl.) (1966): Freud, S. On the History of the Psycho-Analytic Movement. New York: W.W. Norton

Sarteschi, U. (1909): Contributo all'istologia patologica cella presbiofrenia. Rivista sperim. freniatria 35, 464

Schnitzler, J.G. (1911): Zur Abgrenzung der sog. Alzheimerschen Krankheit. Z. Neurol. Psychiatr. 7, 34

Sourander, P., Sjögren, H. (1970): The concept of Alzheimer's diesease and its clinical implications. In: Alzheimer's Disease and Related Conditions. Wolstenholme, G.E.W., O'Connor, M. (eds.). London: Churchill, pp. 11–50

Taylor, J. (1931): Selected Writings of John Hughlings Jackson. New York: Basic Books, pp. 411–421

Tibbitts, C. (1957): Aging in the Modern World. Ann Arbor: University of Michigan

Truman, H.S. (1955): In: Memoirs, Vol. I. Year of Decisions. Garden City: Doubleday

Wilkins, R.H., Brody, I.A. (1969): Alzheimer's Disease. Arch. Neurol. 21, 109–110

2. Clinical Manifestations as a Determinant of Dementia

General Considerations

The terminal phase of the slow inexorable process that disintegrates the human mind results in the most profound form of depravity known to mankind. Physical disability with a variable painful overlay certainly creates widespread sentiment of sympathy. Mental retardation evokes universal grief for a life that could have been. However, the transformation of a viable functioning intellectual animal into a vegetative being without awareness, and without responsiveness represents the ultimate degradation not only for the human but for any other animal species. There is nothing very subtle about its impact; yet it has inspired some of the most poignant poetry and prose every recorded. For example, Shakespeare speaks for King Lear about his mental confusion:

> Does any here know me? This is not Lear:
> Does Lear walk thus? speak thus? Where are his eyes?
> Either his notion weakens, or his discernings
> Are lethargied. Ha! waking? Tis not so.
> Who is it than can tell me who I am?

and finally about the welcome of death:

> Vex not his ghost: O! let him pass; he hates him
> That would upon the rack of this tough world
> Stretch him out longer. (Shakespeare.)

Early clinicians also speak passionately of dementia.

For a man to be absolutely unconscious, or synonymously demented, is for him to have no will, no memory, no reason and no emotion. (Huglings Jackson, 1860.)

The lowest state to which it is possible for a human to sink . . . the shattered wreck of mental organization. (Maudsley, 1868.)

I need scarcely describe senile insanity to you; engraft a little excitement and extra troublesomeness, a few more foolish fancies, and waywardness on the impaired memory gradually increasing, the garrulity passing into childishness, and this second childhood passing more or less rapidly into total fatuity "and mere oblivion sans teeth, sans eyes, sans taste, sans everything", (*As You Like It*) and you will have the disease. (Skae and Clouston, 1873.)

. . . in some cases, apathetic, mindless, without thought or emotion the individual lives on, a mute, almost a motionless vegetating automaton. (H.C. Wood, 1887.)

The natural outcome of the exhaustion of the initial impetus which started the organism upon its course of life and kept it going; the natural expression of that dissipation of energy which accompanies the integration of matter in the process of evolution. It is by this gradual subsidence to rest of the process of storing and expending energy, that life tends to terminate (Mercier, 1905.)

All these writers are declaring a devolution of the human species to a primitive level. However, we should be aware that this is not a regression to childhood, to the level of a primate, or to that of any animal. They are declaring the pathos of a nonintegrated being, who is unaware of its environment, of its requirements for survival, indeed of itself. It is important to realize that this is not merely a loss of higher cortical function, a lack of humaness. We are involved with a loss of an integrative function that is common to all surviving species and enables them to react to environmental stimuli and to enact external responses and thus perpetuate their existence. Most pathetically, the lack of consciousness is unaccompanied by a destruction of the most basic level of integration, that which is essential for the internal maintenance of the organism. So existence continues until some welcome accident terminates the tragedy.

Curiously the onset of this devastation is usually so insidious that only in retrospect can one be certain of such a change. The subtlety of intellectual decline is inherent in a description of early dementia by Roth and Myers (1969):

> The patient is unable to discern common themes or essential differences. He cannot apply experiences to new situations or separate the significant from the trivial. His ideas are meagre and he is unable to grasp new ones.

A comparison with a description of normal aging by Lhermitte and Nicolas (1924) is interesting:

> The outstanding features (of healthy old age) include diminished acuity of memory, or better a loss of adherence to recent events, impaired faculty of rapid evocation of events, loss of fluidity and weakness of creative imagination.

The chief symptom of early dementia is memory loss but practically everyone over 65 confesses to some problem with memory. In most people this defect is not progressive and is of the benign variety described by Kral (1962) as

> . . . an inability to recall on occasion and only temporarily certain relatively unimportant parts of an experience such as a name, date or place while the event, of which the forgotten data form a part can be recalled.

When the event itself cannot be recalled, the memory loss is considered malignant. Certainly this is not a very striking distinction, yet both Kral and Kay et al. (1966) maintain that serious forgetfulness is a most important prognostic indicator not only of organic mental disease but also of premature death. Kral has found that 61.7% of these people died within 4 years while only 38.2% were dead in the benign group. In their 4-year follow-up, Kay et al. noted that memory loss was a more frequent correlate of early death than age.

The difficulty in comparing early dementia with normal aging is the imprecision which is present in every definition of the average elderly person. Despite the decline of IQ after 25, there is no age at which a predictable decline of intelligence will occur in each person. Nonetheless, it is relatively common to observe nondemented elderly who have lost an interest in friends and community, who are not receptive to new ideas, who seem content with minimal activity, and who forget. This is so similar to the first stage of dementia that it forms the clinical basis of the hypothesis that senile dementia is premature or accelerated aging.

When more obvious clinical problems, temporal and spatial disorientation, aphasia, agnosia, apraxia, and seizures occur, the recognition of an impending mental crisis is easy. There has been general recognition that the focal symptoms and seizures have a tendency to occur in younger dements (Sourander and Sjögren, 1968; Lauter and Meyer, 1968). The historical view, that this incidence is an indication of a different disease process (Alzheimer's disease), is no longer considered valid. The final stage of dementia can be associated with either profound apathy with little or no spontaneity or with marked spontaneous hyperactivity. The latter group constitutes the presbyophrenia of the older literature. Fischer (1910) was convinced that there is a selectivity of plaques and tangles for the hyperactive group but this has not been confirmed by subsequent studies. At the present time, the difference in spontaneous activity is not believed to have nosologic significance.

Functional Mental Syndromes as a Manifestation of Brain Disease

The initial occurrence of affective mental problems in old age has always been considered to have some relationship to aging per se, to brain disease (dementia), or to an age-related disorder such as arteriosclerosis. It was very natural to believe that age, nutrition, and circulation combined to cause an involution of the brain (indeed of all organs), which weakened all mental faculties including those related to emotion. Therefore affective disorders occurring in the senium were labeled appropriately as senile melancholia, senile mania, and senile confusion. The implication of these titles was that they represented another aspect of senile brain degeneration and, as such, recovery would never be quite complete, unlike the similar diesease in the young.

Two very evident inconsistencies necessitated qualification of this concept. These included the fact that the respective characters of these disorders were indistinguishable except for age and also that they could be completely cured in the elderly. Notice the ambiguity when Bleuler (1916) wrote discouragingly about this problem:

> The actual senile psychoses, that we know, all have a definite tendency to progress, or expressed anatomically, to the gradual destruction of the brain. That there are not also curable psychoses belonging to senility, is naturally not excluded as yet. But with these I should not like to class "senile melancholias" with mild organic features or organic confusions and deliria, because on closer examination it is always found that after the disappearance of the striking symptoms the patient is, in the sense of dementia senilis, a weakened individual. Therefore, I conceive such storms as intercurrent manifestations of a senile brain degeneration, just as in pronounced senile dementia and analogous to the acute appearances in paresis and schizophrenia, and theoretically I place the major disease in the foreground, even though there are cases where the restoration of equilibrium has practically the significance of a cure.

This was quite different from the optimism of Savage in 1920:

> As far as mental disorders are concerned, I would more hopefully treat a patient who had broken down for the first time at sixty than one who broke down at sixteen.

Another interesting situation developed between the organic concept of aging disorders and the psychoanalysis. We have observed already how Freud's psychoanalytical school dominated psychiatry, particularly after 1910, and generated disregard for organic concepts of grain dysfunction. However, Freudian psychiatry could not cope with mental problems in the aged, since it used abnormal conditioning of the brain during early life as the basis for behavioral disorders. This concept was a perfect explanation of the preponderance of functional disease in young people, but it was hardly satisfactory when applied to the new occurrence in old age. So the organic basis of age-related mental disorder was not questioned during the Freudian era and, actually, a dichotomy between affective disease in the old and in the young became more distinct.

This attitude continued until Post (1951), but more thoroughly Roth (1955), began to question these views. By repetitive follow-up they were able to show that affective psychosis (senile melancholia and mania) and paraphrenia (late-onset schizophrenia) had a distinctly different prognosis than senile dementia and arteriosclerotic dementia. Even more important was the statistical evidence, presented by Roth (1955), that affective psychosis and paraphrenia were curable disorders, just like the functional disease of the young. In 1962, Corsellis provided the pathologic confirmation of this distinction by observing that functional disease was unaccompanied by brain damage in the aged just as it was in the young. These studies stimulated a reconsideration of other aspects of functional disorders in the senium. Does the late onset of functional disease indicate a predisposition for organic disease? Can senile dementia or arteriosclerosis cause functional syndromes?

A predisposition among functional psychotics for organic dementia has been investigated by several groups (Kay et al., 1955; Larson et al., 1963; Post, 1962). The most complete data appears in the study by Kay et al. Of 367 aged psychotics 14 (4%) had both functional and organic syndromes. In only six cases did the functional syndrome precede the organic diesease by a reasonable interval, suggestive of a different mechanism. Their study includes 175 affective psychotics, so a mere 3.3% of the functional group have developed organic dementia. Larson et al. note only 18 of 376 senile dements who had a previous history of psychoneurosis which is almost identical to the findings of Kay et al. Post has found that 7% of his 100 patients with affective disorders developed senile dementia. Since the prevalence of senile dementia in the general population over 65 has generally been stated to be 5%–10% (Kay, 1972) the occurrence of organic degeneration in functional syndromes indicates a susceptibility similar to that for the general population.

Another aspect of this problem is the presence of organic symptoms in a setting of functional psychoses. Memory deficit, confusion, and focal neurologic signs are described in 14% of affective psychotics by Kay et al. and in 19% of Post's group. This appears to be most common among the depressions and undoubtedly has been the cause of gloomy considerations like those of Bleuler. However, the incidence of organic indicators appears to be no different before or after the age of 65. Furthermore, the therapeutic effectiveness is not considered to be affected by the organic symptomatology even in the mixed group where overt dementia was present (Post, 1965).

The evolution of affective psychosis and paraphrenia in organic mental disease is much more difficult to evaluate. Strecker and Ebaugh (1951) state that 16% of their cases had paranoia and 7% had depressed and agitated states. Rothschild (1956) clearly remarks that "the paranoid form of senile psychosis . . . constitutes 20%–25% of all (senile) psychosis". Larson et al. (1963) show 18% of their cases to be of the paranoid type, 10% are of the affective type, and 3% have a combination of both. These studies indicate that 25%–30% of cases of organic dementia have some functional coloring.

A more detailed investigation of this relationship reveals some surprising conclusions, since arteriosclerosis rather than senile dementia has been associated with affective psychosis. Roth (1955) is quite clear when he states:

The incidence of affective symptoms in senile psychosis is low and probably due to chance association. But more than one quarter of arteriosclerotic psychosis have affective symptoms.

Post (1968) concurs with this view:

Senile dementia was only rarely discovered in association with affective illnesses and it also occurred at a later date no more often than might be expected.

Kay et al. (1955) also note this relationship and express the bewilderment caused by this findings:

It is not clear why arteriosclerotic dementia rather than senile psychosis, a common disease, tends to complicate a small proportion of affective disorders of old age. The association of these last two conditions is very uncommon.

An association between late-onset schizophrenia and senile dementia has been affirmed by Kay (1962) and Post (1966), who found a 21% and 22% incidence of patients in whom the organic component had been apparent at the onset of the functional problem. When late-onset schizophrenia is unaccompanied by organic dementia, there is no predisposition to develop an organic syndrome. The schizophrenia itself does not appear to be unique when it is associated with organic disease:

In patients with proven brain pathology all three forms of what some workers would call "symptomatic schizophrenia" were encountered with equal frequency: a simple auditory hallucinosis (especially in association with deafness) a schizophrenic psychosis, but also syndromes characterized by Schneider's First Rank phenomena. Suppression of all types of late schizophrenic symptoms was equally successful in patients with or without cerebral disorders. (Post, 1968.)

These clinical studies have been emphasized because they had a pathologic correlation which was sadly lacking in most surveys of this type. Corsellis (1962), Sourander and Sjögren (1968), and Tomlinson et al. (1970) have all shown that the functional psychotic states are unaccompanied by significant numbers of plaques and tangles. The low incidence of affective psychosis in pure senile dementia has been confirmed by Corsellis (1962), for it occurs in only 6% of this category whereas 20% of the arteriosclerotic group have this problem. Paranoid idealogy appears in 23% and 20% of senile dementia and arteriosclerotic dementia respectively. However, no distinct morphologic change could be observed in the presence of these syndroms. Roth et al. (1968) are very explicit on this point when they try to correlate the quantitative assay of plaques and tangles with functional disease. They concluded that

. . . there was no evidence that degeneration changes had contributed significantly to the causation of illness in patients with functional psychiatric disorders or delirious states.

These studies appear to indicate several conclusions about functional mental disease in the aged. (1) There is no significant difference between an onset before or after the age of 60 either in terms of treatment or as a predisposition for the development of organic brain disease. The higher mortality of the over-60 age group can be related to other age-related causes of death that are more common in the older age group. (2) Both schizophrenia and affective psychoses can occur in a setting of organic brain disease. We must consider the possbility that the brain damage is causing a transmitter imbalance similar to that which evolves independently in functional mental disease. The precise etiologic relationship of organic dementia with schizophrenia and affective disorders has not been clarified.

We have seen that morphology, with the possible exception of multi-infarct dementia, has not revealed an insight into the basis of abnormal personality and behavior. So it is not surprising that, within the last 20 years, a chemical rather than a morphologic explanation has been the prime consideration. It seems appropriate to evaluate these extensive studies, since they may be able to help us explain the difference between senile dementia and arteriosclerosis.

The effectiveness of psychopharmacology in the treatment of affective psychosis and schizophrenia led to an intensive study of the biochemical characteristics of these compounds. These researchers showed that most of these drugs primarily affected the activity of catecholamines, especially noradrenaline. This information led to the catecholamine hypothesis of affective disorders which proposes

> that some, if not all, depressions are associated with an absolute or relative decrease in catecholamines, particularly norepinephrine, available at central adrenergic receptor sites. Elation, conversely, may be associated with an excess of such amines. (Shildkraut, 1965.)

It is important to realize that this theory was formulated entirely on empirical information. The cell biology of the noradrenergic nervous system was derived almost entirely from studies on the peripheral noradrenergic system and the central counterpart was believed to function similarly. The presence of such a system in the brain was demonstrated by transmitter, enzyme, and metabolite assay. Drugs affecting transmitter levels, enzyme activity, and metabolites were recognized to have a pronounced clinical effect upon human affective disorders and could induce behavioral changes in experimental animals. No real information about the physiology of the central noradrenergic system was available.

Within the last 10 years, a vast array of information involving transmitter levels, enzyme activity, and metabolite levels in patients with affective disorders both untreated and treated, has appeared in the medical literature. Much of the early data seemed to support this viewpoint; however, conflicting results and more critical appraisal (Shopsin et al., 1974) resulted in the following conclusion by Moses and Robins (1975):

> Alteration of monoamine metabolism as an etiologic factor in depressive illness remains a possibility if the mechanism involves blocking of the uptake of amines into neurons or changes in membrane permeability. It is unlikely that an alteration of amine metabolism per se is involved, since four selected metabolizing enzymes previously studied showed no difference in activity and the present study shows no depletion of amines.

The disappointment in the failure of the catecholamine hypothesis is comparable to the disillusionment that had accompanied the downfall of plaques and tangles. However, other research of this period has yielded some insight into the anatomy and physiology of the central noradrenergic system. At this time the most definite statement is that it is more complex than the peripheral noradrenergic system. The central noradrenergic system arises chiefly from a limited number of nerve cells in the brain stem but these cells spawn a tremendous network of nerve fibers, which integrate with all levels of the brain (Hartman, 1973). A relatively simple network in the area postrema has dynamics of transmitter turnover comparable to the peripheral noradrenergic system (Torack, 1975). The same transmitter (noradrenaline) can induce excitation or inhibition; it can interact with other transmitter compounds, which now include biogenic amines, amino acids, and amino fatty acids (Reis, 1974). One aspect of this interrelationship has been demonstrated between catecholamines and acetylcholine in several patients with manic symptoms (Janowsky et al., 1972).

Perhaps the most exciting new information about senile dementia is the reduction of choline acetyl transferase (CAT) activity in the cerebral cortex. In three out of six cases Bowen et al. (1976) found about a 50% reduction of activity. This was confirmed by Davies and Maloney (1976) who also noted a similar fall in cholinesterase activity. Perry et al. (1977) also found a very striking 68% reduction of CAT but not in muscarinic cholinergic receptor binding. This seems to indicate a significant reduction of cholinergic neurons in the cortex. The potential of acetylcholine to cause trouble is immense, not only because of a possible link with adrenergic systems, but also because it can be either inhibitory or excitatory depending upon the type of receptor present.

The real significance of psychosyndromes in organic dementia is not known at this time. The contention that they are a manifestation of transmitter imbalance was based upon the widely recognized effectiveness of psychotropic drugs to control these syndromes, especially in the early stages of the disease. This is the only aspect of dementia that is amenable to treatment, so a causal relationship to brain change is debatable. Furthermore, these drugs are equally effective in nondemented patients, so no particular relationship to brain degeneration is implied by these findings. The discovery of CAT loss adds an entirely new dimension to this association. Not only is there real evidence of a transmitter abnormality, but this may be linked to the cause of the problem. Cholinergic neurons seem to participate in the destructive processes of senile dementia (Spillane et al., 1977). This would be a strong argument that the psychosyndromes are an integral part of the clinical presentation of organic dementia and not merely an incidental occurrence.

Acute Confusion

... Any condition of rapidly evolving clouding of consciousness produced by some extraneous cause or appearing for no discernable reason and occurring neither in a setting of definite dementia as far as could be judged from the patient's level of adjustment to the demands of daily life nor as a complication of one of the other diseases defined above. (Affective psychosis, paraphrenia, senile psychosis, arteriosclerotic psychosis.) (Roth, 1955.)

This simple definition summarized a widely recognized mental problem in the aged and established it as a distinct psychiatric syndrome. However, clinical cases of this type were appreciated long ago not because of their sudden onset, but, perhaps more importantly, because some of these people would recover completely. A good example of reversible mental illness was cited by Clouston in 1874:

L. F., 63, a man of a cheerful disposition and somewhat intemperate habits. Three months ago he had an old ulcerated leg healed up. Had a perineal abscess a fortnight ago, which was opened, and since then has been affected in mind. The attack is recent, and came on suddenly. He took fancies that he was rich, got excited, and had a great craving for drink, which he indulged, and became much worse after it. On admission he was greatly exalted, saying he was possessed of all knowledge, power, and wealth. He was excited, shouting and crying, said he was the "Messiah God", that he had millions of money. He did not sleep, and his appetite was poor. He was dirty in his habits, and constantly restless. He was fed well, and got tonics, chiefly iron and quinine. Within a month he was quiet and almost rational and free from delusions. In about three weeks more he began to suffer from headaches, and soon became melancholic and morbidly anxious about his health. After having begun to sleep well, he again lost the power or sleeping in this melancholic stage. In about another month he gradually got out of the depression, and passed into a quietly contented, rational, sane senility. He went home, and ended his days in peace after some years.

Memory loss, temporal and spatial disorientation, hallucination, and occasionally an affective disorder can render this condition indistinguishable from the early stage of senile dementia, but the rapid onset is a strong argument for a different kind of illness.

It was the intention of Roth to establish en entity apart from senile dementia:

> Our hypothesis was that acute confusion whether due to a specific toxic, infective or metabolic factor or to no identifiable cause was a phenomenon distinct from these degenerative diseases.

He found that within a year about 50% of these people were alive and well while the rest were dead. In reality he offered distinction from degenerative disorders in virtue of the high cure rate but he also showed a definite difference from the functional disorders because of the high mortality rate. This dual distinction is intriguing because organic and functional are the only major categories which are recognized. What is acute confusion

As shown by Roth (1955), acute confusion occurs more in females; this differs from arteriosclerosis but is similar to senile dementia. It tends to occur at a younger age than senile dementia, yet it does not have the great incidence between 60 and 69 that is found in affective psychosis and paraphrenia. These cases account for 8.4% of hospital admissions for mental disease, which is about the same percentage as that of paraphrenia and arteriosclerosis. The actual incidence is probably very much higher, because short-lived confusion, 24—48 h in duration, is conceded to be common among the elderly and these people are not usually hospitalized.

A varied etiology was intimated in the original description and this has become very clear subsequently (McCarron and McCormick, 1965). Sjögren (1964) listed eight categories including commotio cerebri, infections, intoxications, pernicious anemia, diabetes mellitus, cardiac disease, postoperative states, and inanition. Recently Libow reported 50 causes of "acute and potentially reversible mental changes; pseudo-senility" and he left out the one which seems to be most common in nursing homes — hip fracture. There is no doubt that a variety of metabolic dysfunctions can cause acute dementia, of which hypothyroidism and hyponatremia are prominent. However, many cases have no distinct cause and are related less tangibly to physical or emotional stress. I say less tangibly, because the stressful situation may be quite evident, but the reaction to stress is very subjective and not easily defined. Kral (1967) has been concerned particularly with this aspect of the problem but specific effects of stress on nerve cells or, more important, certain parts of the brain are completely unappreciated at this time.

Both Kral (1973) and Roth (1955) state that full recovery can be expected in about 50% of hospitalized cases of acute confusion. However, these authors differ upon the fate of the less fortunate other half. Roth states that 80% of these patients will die in 6 months and within a year all will be dead. On the other hand Kral remarks:

> of the remaining 50% about half die. A clinical picture not distinguishable from senile dementia develops in the others.

There seems to be little doubt that those people who die within a year do so because of the severity of the underlying disease process. However there are some patients who do not improve, who survive more than a year, and who become indistinguishable from senile dementia patients.

The medical literature does not appear to contain an autopsy report on a case of acute confusion. Sjögren (1964) reports that neuropathologic examination was done in 27 cases but they are lumped with 33 cases of functional disease and not analyzed as a group. Avery (1945) states that 8 of 17 cases of confusion suffered from a typical dementia and died but there is no description of brain pathology. Lowenberg and Rothschild (1931) describe a case of sudden-onset dementia in a 37-year-old woman who had numerous plaques when she died at 47. Jansens' (1911) report of Alzheimer's disease (AD) in a man of 53 started with acute delirium. Goodman (1953) claims that three of his cases of AD had a sudden onset of mental symptoms following surgical procedures. However, in none of these is an acute confusional episode defined as such in the clinical protocol.

The following case report is an illustration of what can happen in a person who does not return to normal.

G. M., a 75-year-old white female, was hospitalized for the first time with acute confusion that occurred during a telephone conversation with her son. Apparently there was no loss of consciousness, no obvious paralysis (she answered the door easily) but she appeared confused and, while she could speak, she had difficulty putting words together meaningfully. An EEG showed diffuse slow activity of moderately high voltage. Electrolytes were depressed, Na − 118, K − 3.1, Cl − 82. EKG was normal. The electrolytes were finally corrected 6 days after admission and the next day her mental status was described as improved. This seemed to be a case of mental confusion due to hyponatremia. She was discharged 9 days after admission.

However, she never returned to the mental clarity she had prior to this time. Four months later, she was rehospitalized because of an aggravated confusion. Again she improved and was discharged. For the next 3 years, she was able to maintain her own apartment in a retirement complex that provided maid service, dining facilities, and health service. More or less constant complaints during this period included forgetting if she had eaten earlier, losing her way back to her room, and a lack of money for her bills (she was economically affluent). There was a depressive episode about midway in this interval, which cleared with parmacotherapy. Otherwise there appeared to be a slowly progressive mental disorder, which prompted her transfer to a nursing home after 3 years.

The next 1.5 years represent a continuation of the slow progression of the previous 3 years. However, at the end of that interval, another hospitalization was prompted by a complaint of numbness in the left arm. At this time a CCT scan revealed brain atrophy. An EEG was reported as "diffuse slow dysthythmia which may relate to diffuse metabolic or organic loss". Somewhat improved, she returned to the nursing home, where a more rapid proggression of mental decline was noted. She developed paranoid idealogy, incontinence of urine, an inability to feed herself, and complete disorientation to time and place. She has no interest in her surroundings or herself. Apart from the nature of its onset, this would seem to be a classic history of senile dementia.

The impressive aspect of acute confusion is its sudden dramatic onset, its relationship to recognizable body disease, and the distinct possibility of complete recovery. Not only is this condition different from other categories of mental diesease in the aged, it is also quite distinct from aging itself. Aging must be considered to be endogenous disease. But this condition occurs because some influence outside of the brain is causing the brain dysfunction. Its prevalence in the old-age period must indicate that the aging brain is more susceptible, since many of the defined causes are not unique to age.

A most important consideration is the evolution of a chronic brain syndrome indistinguishable from senile dementia. This emphasizes the urgency to identify the cause of the problem, to cure it, and to maintain adequate control. One could speculate that my case with the recurring hyponatremia could have been prevented by more effective control. There seems to be little doubt that this condition has evolved to brain atrophy. The lack of pathologic reports on this matter suggests that no distinctive abnormality is present. Tomlinson (1971), who examined the brains of Roth's patients, reports that 4 out of 50 dements have insufficient senile plaques or vascular disease to explain the dementia. But there is no indication that these people have chronic confusion. This lack of knowledge is even more perplexing when we consider that acute confusion is the only dementing syndrome that is reversible.

Specialized Syndromes in Dementia

Creutzfeldt-Jakob Disease

A more rapid progression of dementia (2 months to 2 years) and the addition of motor symptoms have been considered the major clinical distinctions of Creutzfeldt-Jakob disease (CJD). However, within this rather broad definition several patterns of neurologic syndromes have been characterized sufficiently to suggest various forms of this disorder. In CJD a distinctive neuronal degeneration occurs so that clinicopathologic correlation is quite uncomplicated. Moreover since the disease has been transmitted to chimpanzees, this is one dementia for which an etiologic agent is recognized. So at least in this case the significance of distinctive clinical syndromes can be evaluated using both pathologic and etiologic criteria.

The original description by Creutzfeldt in 1920 and the subsequent cases reported by Jakob emphasized motor involvement (spastic pseudosclerosis), myoclonus, pyramidal symptoms, and the fulminating dementia. However, in 1928 Heidenhain noted a visual agnosia with prominent pathologic change in the occipital lobe and suggested that these were different from the case of Creutzfeldt and Jakob. Somewhat later Jones and Nevin (1954) reported a distinctive EEG in these visuooccipital variants plus a prominent status spongiosis which prompted a proposed category of subacute spongiform encephalopathy.

Siedler and Malamud (1963) disagreed with this concept and argued instead for a distinction based upon regional involvement. They gathered together 15 cases of their own and added 57 from the literature to evaluate clinicopathologic distinction. They decided that the neuronal changes, the sponginess, and the gliosis offered no basis for separation. Rather they felt that the distribution of these changes could be associated with various clinical syndromes. So they established four forms, which they termed (1) cortical, (2) cortical striatal, (3) cortical spinal, and (4) corticostriato spinal. Two years later, Brownell and Oppenheimer (1965) added a corticostriatal cerebellar form and more recently Krucke et al. (1973) described cases of paleoencephalic involvement that looked like kuru.

Kuru is a dementing disease of Fore tribesmen in New Guinea. The localized incidence and the cannibalism of the tribe suggested an infectious etiology. A cell-free extract of kuru brain was used for transmission to animals and it was successfully completed in 1966 by Gajdusek et al. The infectious agent was called a virus because of its size (as determined by passage through a filter) and a slow virus because the inoculated primates did not become ill until an average 14 months later. Transmission of CJD was attempted because of the pathologic similarity between CJD and kuru (Klatzko et al., 1959). The transmission of CJD to a chimpanzee was reported by Gibbs et al. in 1969.

At the time of this writing 68 cases of CJD have been transmitted to a variety of laboratory animals, chiefly chimpanzees and monkeys. Only 8 cases have been considered nontransmissible, which means that the animal has no clinical or pathologic evidence of disease after 4 years. This is unlike kuru, which is 100% transmissible. Therefore the cases that transmit have been termed transmissible viral dementia (TVD) to distinguish them from CJD, which does not transmit. A single agent (TVD agent) has been thought to cause the animal disease, since no species susceptibility or characteristic incubation time can be related to any of the diagnostic categories. The details of the transmission studies will be discussed in the chapter on slow virus disease.

The clinical characteristics of the first 12 cases of TVD were reviewed by Roos et al. (1973) and the first 56 cases were evaluated by Traub et al. (1977). Only two characteristics of the TVD group were significantly different from the nontransmissible group (Table 2.1). The first involved an average duration of the dementing syndrome in TVD which was 8.0 ± 9.3 months while that of the other cases was 23.4 ± 27.1 months. The second distinction of TVD is the higher incidence of a characteristic EEG. So the appearance of the different neurologic patterns (cortical, corticostriatal, etc.) has no significance as an indicator of transmissibility at this time.

Table 2.1 Clinical and pathologic characteristics of TVD, nontransmitted CJD, and untransmissible CJD (after Traub et al., 1977)

Characteristic	TVD	Nontransmitted CJD	Untransmissible CJD	All TVD and CJD
Number of patients	56	70	8	126
Males	28	41	4	69
Females	28	29	4	57
Males/females	1.00	1.41	1.00	1.21
Range age of onset (yrs.)	34−78	26−74	38−68	26−78
Average age of onset (yrs.)	56.3 ± 9.5	55.7 ± 11.2	20.5 ± 9.2	56.0
Range of duration (months)	1.5 − 68	2 − 72	3 − 72	1.5 − 72
Average duration (months)	8.0 ± 9.3	12.1 ± 14.8	23.4 ± 27.1	10.3
Behavioral disturbance	28/54 (52%)	26/60 (43%)	5/8 (63%)	54/114 (47%)
Higher cortical dysfunction	30/54 (56%)	36/62 (58%)	6/8 (75%)	67/116 (58%)
Upper motor neuron signs	43/55 (78%)	44/61 (72%)	7/8 (88%)	88/116 (76%)
Lower motor neuron signs	14/53 (26%)	20/36 (56%)	3/8 (38%)	34/ 89 (38%)
Basal ganglia disorder	29/54 (54%)	35/64 (55%)	2/8 (25%)	64/118 (54%)
Myoclonus	48/54 (89%)	50/63 (79%)	6/8 (75%)	98/117 (84%)
Cerebellar dysfunction	35/53 (66%)	39/62 (63%)	3/8 (38%)	74/115 (64%)
Visual disturbance	24/54 (44%)	23/59 (39%)	4/8 (50%)	47/113 (42%)
Characteristic EEG	36/53 (70%)	26/57 (46%)	4/8 (50%)	63/110 (57%)
Seizures	11/53 (21%)	17/60 (28%)	3/8 (38%)	28/113 (25%)
Neuronal vacuolation	51/52 (98%)	64/67 (96%)	8/8 (100%)	116/119 (98%)
Neurofibrillary tangles	5/51 (10%)	5/62 (8%)	2/8 (25%)	10/113 (9%)
Amyloid plaques	6/51 (12%)	10/62 (16%)	2/8 (25%)	16/113 (14%)
Family history [a]	7/56 (13%)	4/70 (6%)	1/8 (13%)	11/126 (9%)

[a] Of disease suggestive of, or confimed as, CJD.

Some further discussion of motor neuron involvement and myoclonus appears desirable. This type of involvement has been used widely to distinguish CJD from AD because of its frequent presence in CJD. However, infrequent, myoclonus has been recognized in AD and 13 cases have been reviewed by Jakob (1968). The usefulness of myoclonus as indicator of transmissibility has not been revealed to date. Traub et al. have found no difference in the occurrence of upper or lower neuron signs, extrapyramidal involvement and myoclonus among the cases that do or do not transmit. Actually the appearance of myoclonus can prompt a change in the diagnosis from AD to CJD. An example of this problem can be seen in the following case taken from the files of C.J. Gibbs Jr. (1976).

A 51-year-old white male had a 5-year history of slowly progressive dementia. Four years after the onset of distinct memory loss and confusion he developed seizures, which were followed by generalized myoclonic jerks. This rapid decline was believed to be compatible with CJD or a brain tumor. A cerebral biopsy revealed senile plaques (SP) and an occasional neurofibrillary tangle (NF). Animal transmission was attempted but it was without result 5 years later.

A current evaluation of TVD would indicate a repidly progressive dementia, preferably with myoclonus, a characteristic EEG, and a duration of less than 1 year. Although the various clinical syndromes seem to offer no basis for distinction, a most consistent feature of the pathology is neuronal vacuolation in the cortex. The one case of TVD without vacuolation is a case of hereditary AD. So the entity should be considered to be cortical disease plus a variety of other brain involvement. Undoubtedly this is related to the presence of a characteristic EEG in 70% of the cases.

Klüver-Bucy Syndrome (Limbic Encephalitis)

Dementia has been conceived of chiefly as a disorder of the neocortex but AD as well as subacute dementia is known to have basal ganglionic (Pearce, 1974), cerebellar (Worster-Drought et al., 1944), and motor system (Jacob, 1968) involvement. In particular, extrapyramidal features of the Parkinsonian type have been reported recently in 40 of 65 unselected patients with organic dementia (Pearce, 1974). Such diffuse clinical involvement complicates the concept that AD is a system disease only of the neocortex. Actually, even Hughlings Jackson said that dementia was a loss of all four of his levels of consciousness, not just the highest one.

Our current understanding of brain organization has progressed quite a bit from Hughlings Jackson and generally three levels of integration are recognized (MacLean, 1970; Yakovlev, 1948). The neocortex (ectopallium) is the most recent part of the brain, reaching its highest development in man. The limbic system (mesopallium) has been considered a postreptilian evolution and its more primitive function may be seen in its very intimate association with the olfactory bulb. The lowest level of integration is the reticular system (entopallium), which exists in man chiefly as a regulatory system of body organs other than striated muscle tissue.

The location of each part can be very well appreciated in Yakovlev's diagrams (Figs. 2.1 and 2.2) but the functional role of each system has been more difficult to appreciate. Actually the problem mainly involves the limbic system, since comparative neurology, quite clearly, has linked the reticular system with visceration and the neocortex with intellection. In 1933, Papez had introduced the novel concept that the limbic system is the regulator of emotion. By 1948, this idea had become expanded to a network which controls all forms of expression (Yakovlev). MacLean (1970) has defined six different types of behavior that emanate from the limbic system: searching, aggressive, protective, dejected, gratulant, and caressive.

The action of these three brains has been described most deftly by Yakovlev:

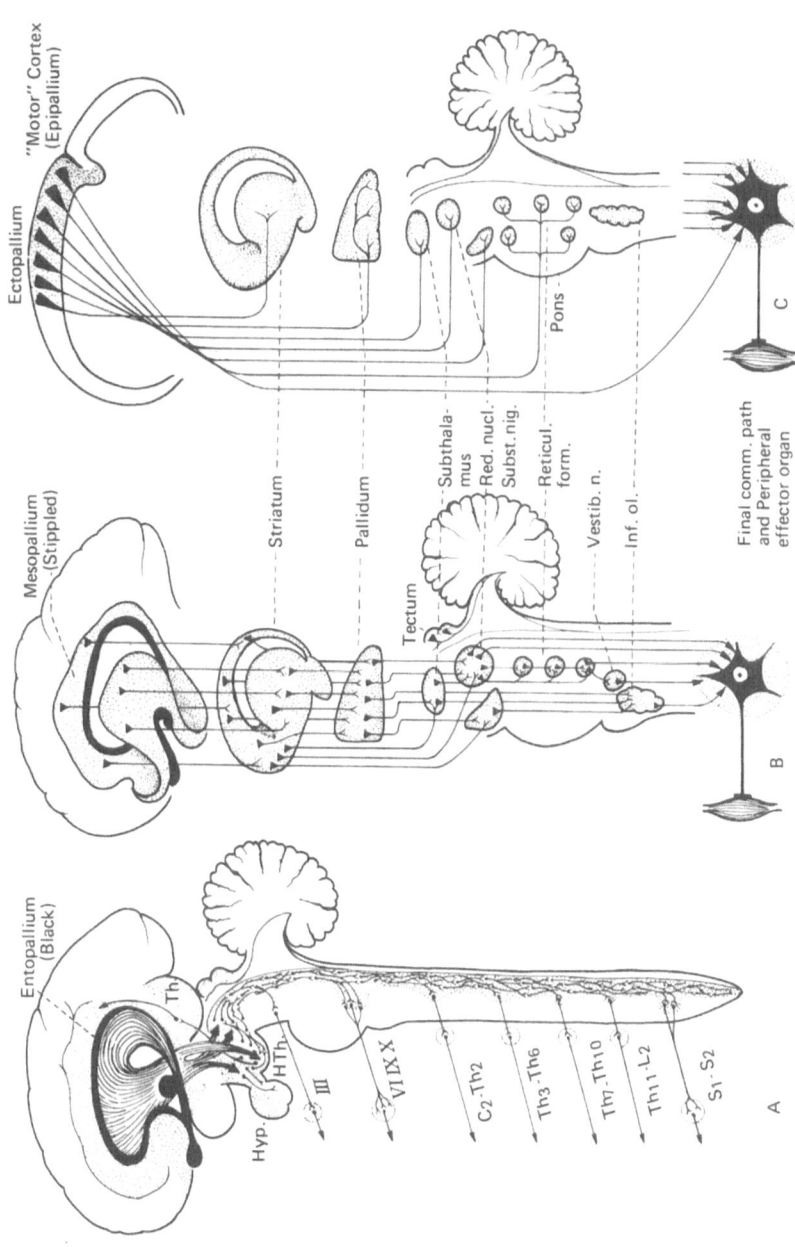

Fig. 2.1. Organization of the brain. (From P.I. Yakovlev.) (A) Innermost system of visceration; (B) intermediate system of expression; (C) outermost system of effectuation

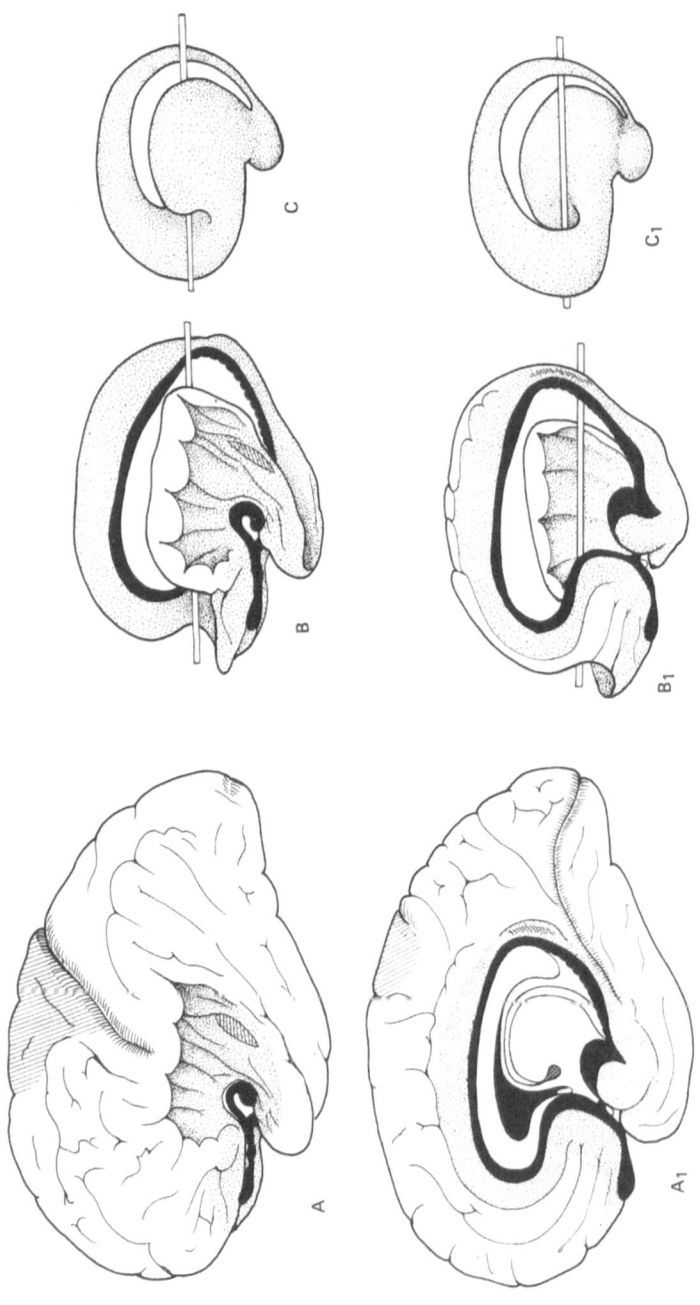

Fig. 2.2. The structural components of three different levels of brain function. (From P.I. Yakovlev.) (A) and (A$_1$) Lateral view of the left and medial view of the right hemispheres (redrawn and modified from C. v. Economo and G. Koskinas). Entopallium – black; mesopallium – stippled; extopallium ("motor" and "premotor" cortex) – vertical lines; specific "sensory" projections – horizontal streaks. (B) and (B$_1$) Mesopallia of the left and right hemispheres dissected. (C) and (C$_1$) Corpora striata, including amygdalae of the left and right hemispheres dissected

1. The sphere of *visceral motility,* such as to and from movement of atoms in tissue and cell metabolism, respiration, circulation, incretion, peristalsis, secretion, excretion and like movements, largely within the body.

2. The sphere of motility of the *outward expression of internal states,* such as hunger, thirst, fear, rage, pleasure, grief, pain and the gamut of the so called emotions, literally e(x) motions, i.e., internal motions brought out – the motor expressions of which – such as facial mimicry, vocalizations, body attitudes and postures – affect the animal but, per se, effect no change in the world of matter about it.

3. The sphere of *motility of effectuation* which creates changes in the world of matter about the animal, i.e., produces work through which the animal impresses itself upon the world of matter, e.g. locomotes, shapes and handles matter, using his own body and parts of it as tools.

It is quite obvious that these functions must interact but the problem is how. A most reasonable hypothesis is that as each new part evolved it became integrated with the part that existed before it. In this way a linkage in series is effected. The important part of this scheme is that real function of a lower level can affect the function of a higher level or levels. So that disease of the limbic system can affect the neocortex. This possibility appears worthy of further study.

In the human brain the limbic system is a diffuse system with some well-recognized components among which are the hippocampus, the hippocampal gyrus, the amygdaloid nucleus, the median forebrain bundle, the septum pellucidum, and the cingulate gyrus. These structures have widespread connections with the rest of the brain, particularly the anterior thalamus and the frontal lobes (Nauta, 1962). The latter is of most interest, because frontal lobe atrophy is the most conspicuous neocortical abnormality in AD.

Our current appreciation of the clinical manifestation of limbic dysfunction is the result of ablation experiments in animals and a study of human diseases that destroy the limbic system. The ablation studies have been evaluated most extensively by Klüver and Bucy between 1937 and 1939. They involve a surgical removal of the amygdala, hippocampus, uncus, and hippocampal gyrus bilaterally, which causes a series of symptoms, populary known as the Klüver-Bucy Syndrome:

Visual "agnosia". Although the animal exhibits no, or at least no gross, defects in its ability to discriminate visually, it appears to have lost the ability to recognize and detect the meaning of animate and inanimate objects on the basis of visual criteria alone. It seems that it can no longer rely on visual cues for detecting that an object is "edible" or "dangerous". Furthermore, a study of the behavior alterations suggests the presence of "agnosic" symptoms in the auditory and tactile fields.

Oral tendencies. There is an extremely strong tendency to examine all objects by mouth. Such an oral examination generally consists of putting the object into the mouth, licking, biting, chewing, touching with the lips and "smelling". There are also strong oral tendencies in that the monkey, instead for picking up objects, tends to contact objects, or parts of them, directly by mouth.

"Hypermetamorphosis" (in the sense of Wernicke). There is a very marked tendency to take notice of an attend to every visual stimulus. Moreover, the animal, as if under the influence of some "irresistible" impulse, tends to touch every object in sight. Noticing an object and performing the necessary motor reactions for contacting it often seem to be a continuous process.

Changes in emotional behavior. There is a diminution, or even a complete absence, of emotional responses in the sense that there are no, or practically no, stimuli capable of eliciting the motor, vocal, and other forms of behavior that are generally associated with anger and fear reactions. Without hesitation the monkey approaches every animate or inanimate object, even live snakes or objects which previous to the operation called forth extreme excitement, avoidance reactions, or other forms of emotional behavior. The facial "expressions" of emotions are often entirely lost.

Changes in sexual behavior. There is a striking increase in sexual activities and in the diversity of sexual manifestations. This hypersexuality which generally appears for the first time several weeks after the operation is exhibited not only when the monkey is caged with other animals, but also when left alone. Various forms of heterosexual, homosexual and autosexual behavior rarely or never seen in normal monkeys can be observed almost continuously or at least at frequent intervals;

an intensification of sexual responses may even be found in castrates and pseudohermaphrodites. Females may show a complete lack of maternal behavior.

Changes in dietary habits. Following the operation the monkey will accept and eat large quantities of ham, bacon, ground beef, broiled lamb chops, smoked whitefish and other kinds of meat offered. Normal rhesus monkeys are generally frugivorous and do not even touch meat when it is offered to them. Furthermore, there may be a striking increase in appetite and food concumption. (Klüver, 1958.)

The human diseases that have shown a predilection for the limbic system are chiefly of known suspected infectious etiology (Brierly et al., 1960; Rose and Symonds, 1960). Most prominent in this groups is the necrotizing encephalitis produced by herpes simplex (Drachman and Adams, 1962). Bilateral temporal lobe involvement is a consistent pattern in simplex encephalitis, which cannot be explained by a unique vasculature or by a spread from contiguous structures. More complete destruction of the limbic system is quite rare but this has been noted in at least two instances (Gascon and Gilles, 1973; Friedman and Allen, 1969). In both of these, a clinical syndrome remarkably similar to the Klüver-Bucy syndrome has been observed in a background of dementia. Symptoms of focal cortical dysfunction, aphasia, agnosia, and apraxia were absent, but otherwise these patients have amnestic syndromes and behavioral disturbance notably similar to AD.

The limbic involvement in encephalitis associated with carcinoma (Corsellis, 1968) and in the more recent report of subacute dementia resembling kuru (Krücke et al., 1973) represents conditions of suspected but unproven viral etiology. In his study, Corsellis had been prompted to suggest that a demented condition could be a development of limbic disease. A detailed clinical report is not presented by Krücke et al., but the distribution of the lesions is so similar to those of Gascon and Gilles that one would suspect that a Klüver-Bucy syndrome had been present in this case. A Klüver-Bucy syndrome in man has also been reported in a male epileptic who had extensive bilateral anterior temporal lobectomy as treatment for his seizures (Terzian and Ore, 1955). More restricted surgery results only in memory loss without personality change (Scoville and Milner, 1957).

Summarily, destruction of the limbic system causes many of the clinical symptoms that are present in dementing syndromes. Inasmuch as focal cortical dysfunction is not present, some additonal component of neocortical disease seems to occur in such dementias as AD. None the less, limbic involvement is suggested early in these conditions by the amnestic syndrome and late in the disease by the changes in expressiveness. Sourander and Sjögren (1968) report that most of their Alzheimer cases showed all the symptoms of the syndrome except abnormal sexual behavior. Pilleri (1966) and Jelgersma (1964) have also commented upon this association. The pathologic changes in the limbic system in AD have been emphaiszed in recent studies by Hooper and Vogel (1976) and by Brun and Gustafson (1976). Some modification of the concept that AD is neocortical disease appears to be indicated by all of these observations.

Normal Pressure Hydrocephalus

The clinical syndrome that Adams et al. (1965) described in relation to enlarged ventricles and normal cerebrospinal fluid (CSF) pressure (Hakim and Adams, 1965) was unique mainly because it was reversible following the installation of a ventricular shunt. Actually, occult or compensated hydrocephalus had been reported earlier (McHugh,

1964) but the dementing syndrome and the reversibility by shunt therapy was not emphasized. After 1965, the effect upon the dementia was stressed and the criteria for shunting were expanded to include AD, since enlarged ventricles also occurred. However, unlike AD, the early cases of normal pressure hydrocephalus (NPH) did not have cortical atrophy or plaques and tangles. Similar effectiveness of shunt therapy was not forthcoming in these cases and the enthusiam for shunt therapy has waned considerably (Messert and Wannamaker, 1974). There evolved some concern that NPH was not a distinct entity but merely a variant of other dementing disease such as AD (Coblentz et al., 1973).

Case Report: I. O., a 77-year-old white male lawyer continued to be active in his law practice until 9 months prior to his hospitalization for shunt therapy. One month later, a Florida vacation was cancelled because of diminished enthusiasm, which accompanied a generalized unresponsiveness and increasing apathy. Two months later, urinary and occasionally fecal incontinence was noted. At this time, a business associate noted reduced ideation and spontaneity of physical activity. Two months prior to surgery he developed gait and hand apraxia. In retrospect, gait apraxia may have been present earlier but was masked by the reduction of physical activity. He had not distinct memory defect until 1 week prior to admission, at which time it appeared virtually complete for recent events.

Within 1 week after the shunt surgery his memory problem seemed to have disappeared. His gait returned to normal within a month. The hand apraxia and incotinence resolved 6 weeks following surgery. Since that time he has returned to his business activity and, while his participation was not at its former level, he has spent 3–4 days a week in his office. At present, it has been 3 months since the shunt was installed.

This case demonstrates all of the original components of the NPH syndrome, "mild impairment of memory, slowness and paucity of thought and action, unsteadiness of gait and urinary incontinence" (Ojemann et al., 1969). The dramatic reversal was actually noted by his wife within 3 days following the placement of the shunt. The relative early occurrence of fecal incontinence and hand apraxia were minor distinctive features of this case. Perhaps more important aspects were the relatively short course (9 months) and the evolving symptomatology at the time of surgery.

After the effectiveness of shunt therapy had been recognized (Adams et al., 1965) CSF dynamics were studied more thoroughly in these patients. A distinct reduction of CSF flow was demonstrated by cisternography using a radioactive tracer, either labeled albumen or indium. The altered CSF dynamics were indicated by a reflux of the tracer into the ventricles but even more by the presence of an obstruction to flow either at the incisura (midbrain) or at some point overlying the cerebral convexities. Because of the normal CSF pressure, this condition was considered to represent a compensated form of obstructive hydrocephalus (Lorenzo et al., 1974). This theory was supported by the work of James et al. (1973), who showed that an obstruction at the level of the incisura in dogs produced ventricular dilatation and elevated pressure for about 60 days, whereupon the pressure returned to normal levels.

The clinical presentation is quite unique because the amnestic syndrome frequently is not an early finding, there are usually no symptoms of neocortical involvement, and the appearance of urinary incontinence is an early event (Messert and Baker, 1966). In typical AD, the apathy usually follows a clear-cut memory loss and disorientation, gait disturbance is usually present only in the terminal stage and may never occur, and incontinence is common only when a complete disregard for self has occurred. These differences in the clinical syndrome appear to justify a contention that this is not some variant of AD.

The sources of this confusion are multiple: (1) AD frequently has meningeal fibrosis and dilated ventricles; (2) abnormal CSF dynamics have been observed in AD (Coblentz et al., 1973); (3) several cases of NPH have been shown to have cortical atrophy with plaques and tangles (Sohn et al., 1973; Coblentz et al., 1973). In AD, the ventricular dilatation has always been considered to follow cerebral atrophy (hydrocephalus ex vacuo) and therefore, this is not an early event. The occurrence of plaques and tangles with altered CSF flow may have several explanations. Many of these cases occur in the seventh and eighth decade when plaques and tangles are found increasingly in the normal aged, so the condition may be present concurrently. Moreover, the meningeal fibrosis of AD may cause a subarachnoid obstruction, so that a component of NPH may be present in some cases. This element of obstruction may be the explanation for the reports of improvement following shunt installation in AD (Shenkin et al., 1973).

The mechanism of brain disease in obstructive hydrocephalus is believed to be an altered equilibrium between parenchymal fluid and CSF at the ependymal interface (Milhorat, 1972). Following an elevation of CSF pressure, the normal flow of fluid from brain to ventricles is reversed so that a stagnation and then an input of fluid into the periventricular extracellular spaces is present (Milhorat, 1972; Strecker et al., 1974). This hydration of periventricular tissue causes demyelination of neighboring axons with nerve dysfunction and ultimate destruction (Weller and Wisniewski, 1969). The part of the brain that assumes the brunt of this injury is not the ectopallium (neocortex) or the mesopallium (limbic system) but the entopallium (reticular system), which is the most primitive part of the brain (see Yakovlev's diagram). Therefore NPH would appear to be a primary dysfunction of the reticular formation. In this context the absence of focal cortical dysfunction, the later onset of an amnestic syndrome, and the early appearance of devisceration (urinary incontinence) become very understandable clinical characteristics.

Summary of Specialized Syndromes

A most important consequence of Yakovlev's "three spheres of brain function" and MacLean's "triune brain" is that the mind is the product of integration at all levels. Then dementia can be a manifestation of disease at each level, if it disrupts this integration. In reality, CJD does seem to be primarily cortical dementia. NPH quite obviously is not cortical dementia; it is entopallial or reticular dementia. AD is confusing because it begins and ends as limbic dementia but, in between, there is cortical dysfunction. Clinical symptoms alone do not appear sufficient to resolve this problem.

Summary of Clinical Manifestations

There seems to be no question regarding the similarity of the early stage of AD to some aspects of normal mental aging, particularly memory loss. In this regard a "malignant memory loss" may have predictive value of subsequent dementia. This seems to indicate an early involvement of the limbic system, which also appears to be vulnerable to an aging process and viral infection. A syndrome of abnormal mental behavior and expressiveness can occur in these early phases and probably indicates a more generalized dysfunction of this system. These conditions resemble functional mental disease and probably would have a similar biochemical correlate.

The evolution of aphasia, agnosia, and apraxia signify an additon of cortical disease. These symptoms have never been considered to be a part of normal aging and they may be present in vascular disease or in CJD, both of which have prominent cortical involvement. Finally, an end stage occurs which can include a Klüver-Bucy syndrome (limbic diesease) of incontinence with paucity of thought and movement, and is similar to NPH. NPH seems to occur as a consequence of meningeal fibrosis.

It is apparent that practically no etiologic agent can be excluded by the clinical aspects of the problem. Normal aging can be indistinguishable from early dementia. Functional mental syndromes seem to be biochemical (transmitter) abnormalities but the precise defects remain to be clarified. Certain viruses (Herpes) have a predilection for the limbic system and an unidentified slow virus is implicated in CJD. Vascular disease can cause focal cortical syndromes and dementia after multiple infarcts is unquestionable. Vascular disease (hemorrhage) and infection can also cause meningeal obstruction and NPH.

Perhaps the most neglected clinical syndrome is acute confusion. Here is a dementia in which the cause frequently is apparent, and in which the process is reversible, at least in 50% of the cases. Paradoxically, if it does not reverse, it can result in a clinical state indistinguishable from terminal AD. I believe that more detailed clinical study is needed, especially of metabolites in the CSF and, above all, it is time to establish some pathologic correlation, even if the brain is normal.

References

Adams, R.D., Fisher, C.M., Hakim, S., Ojemann, R.G., Sweet, W.H. (1965): Symptomatic occult hydrocephalus with normal cerebrospinal fluid pressure. N. Engl. J. Med. 273, 117–126

Avery, L. (1945): Common factors precipitating mental symptoms in the aged. Arch. Neurol. Psychiatry 54, 312–314

Bleuler, E. (1924): Textbook of Psychiatry. (Translated by A.A. Brill). New York: MacMillan, p. 277

Bowen, D.M., Smith, C.B., White, P., Davison, A.N. (1976): Neurotransmitter-related enzymes and indices of hypoxia in senile dementia and other abiotrophies. Brain 99, 459–496

Brierly, J.B., Corsellis, J.A.N., Hierons, R., Nevin, S. (1960): Subacute encephalitis of later adult life mainly affecting the limbic areas. Brain 83, 357–368

Brownell, B., Oppenheimer, D.R. (1965): An ataxic form of subacute presenile polioencephalopathy (Creutzfeldt-Jakob disease). J. Neurol. Neurosurg. Psychiatry 25, 350–361

Brun, A., Gustafson, L. (1976): Distribution of cerebral degeneration in Alzheimer's disease. Arch. Psychiatr. Nervenkr. 223, 15–33

Clouston, T.S. (1884): Clinical Lectures on Mental Disease. Philadelphia: Leas and Son

Clouston, T.S. (1911): Unsoundness of Mind. New York: Dutton

Coblentz, J.M., Mattis, S., Zingesser, L.H., Kasoff, E.S., Wisnieski, H.M., Katzman, R. (1973): Presenile dementia. Arch. Neurol. 29, 299–308

Corsellis, J.A.N. (1962): Mental Illness and the Aging Brain. London: Oxford

Corsellis, J.A.N., Goldberg, G.J., Norton, A.R. (1968): Limbic encephalitis and its association with carcinoma. Brain 91, 481–496

Creutzfeldt, H.G. (1920): Über eine eigenartige herdförmige Erkrankung des Zentralnervensystems. Z. Neurol. Psychiatr. 57, 1–18

Davies, P., Maloney, A.J.F. (1976): Selective loss of central cholinergic neurons in Alheimer's disease. Lancet 2, 1403

Drachman, D.A., Adams, R.D. (1962): Herpes simplex and acute inclusionbody encephalitis. Arch. Neurol. 7, 45–63

Fischer, O. (1910): Die presbyophrene Demenz, deren anatomische Grundlage und klinische Abgrenzung. Z. Neurol. Psychiatr. 3, 371–471

Friedman, H.M., Allen, N. (1969): Chronic effects of complete limbic lobe destruction in man. Neurology 19, 679–690

Gajdusek, D.C., Gibbs, C.J., Jr., Alpers, M. (1966): Experimental transmission of Kuru-like syndrome to chimpanzees. Nature 209, 794–796

Gascon, G.G., Gilles, F. (1973): Limbic dementia. J. Neurol. Neurosurg. Psychiatry 36, 421–430

Gibbs, C.J., Jr., Gajdusek, D.C., Asher, D.M., Alpers, M.P., Beck, E., Daniel, P.M., Matthews, W.B. (1968): Creutzfeldt-Jakob disease (spongiform encephalopathy): transmission to the chimpanzee. Science 161, 388–389

Gibbs, C.J., Jr. (1976): Personal Communication

Goodman, L. (1953): Alzheimer's disease. A clinico-pathologic analysis of twenty-three cases with a theory on pathogenesis. J. Nerv. Ment. Dis. 118, 97–130

Hakim, S., Adams, R.D. (1965): The special clinical problem of symptomatic hydrocephalus with normal cerebrospinal fluid pressure: observations on cerebrospinal fluid hydrodynamics. J. Neurol. Sci. 2, 307–327

Hartman, B.K. (1973): Immunofluorescence of dopamine-beta-hydroxylase. Application of improved methodology to the localization of the peripheral and central noradrenergic nervous system. J. Histochem. Cytochem. 21, 312–332

Heidenhain, A. (1928): Klinische und anatomische Untersuchungen über eine eigenartige organische Erkrankung des Zentralnervensystems im Präsenium. Z. Neurol. Psychiatr. 118, 49–114

Hooper, M.W., Vogel, F.S. (1976): The limbic system in Alzheimer's disease. Am. J. Pathol. 85, 1–13

Jacob, H. (1970): Muscular twitchings in Alzheimer's disease. In: Alzheimer's Disease and Related Conditions. Wolstenholme, G.E.W., O'Connor, M.E. (eds.). London: Churchill, pp. 75–89

Jakob, A. (1921): Über eigenartige Erkrankungen des Zentralnervensystems mit bemerkenswerten anatomischen Befunden. Z. Neurol. Psychiatr. 64, 147–228

James, A.E., Strecker, E.P., Novak, G.R. (1973): Correlation of serial cisternograms and cerebrospinal fluid pressure measurements in experimental communicating hydrocephalus. Neurlogy 23, 1226–1233

Janowsky, D.S., Khaled, El-Sousef M., Davis, J.M., Hubbard, B., Sekerke, H.J. (1972): Cholinergic reversal of manic symptoms. Lancet 1, 1236–1237

Jansone, G. (1911): Ein Fall der Alzheimerschen Krankheit. Cas. Beitr. Psych. Neurol. Bladen 4 and 5

Jelgersma, H.C. (1964): Ein Fall von juveniler hereditärer Demenz vom Alzheimer-Typ mit Parkinsonismus und Klüver-Bucy-Syndrom. Arch. Psychiatr. Nervenkr. 205, 262–266

Jones, D.P., Nevin, S. (1954): Rapidly progressive cerebral degeneration (subacute vascular encephalopathy) with mental disorder, focal disturbances and myoclonic epilepsy. J. Neurol. Neurosurg. Psychiatry 17, 148–159

Kay, D.W.K., Roth, M., Hopkins, B. (1955): Affective disorders arising in the senium 1. Their association with organic cerebral degeneration. J. Ment. Sci. 101, 302–316

Kay, D.W.K.(1962): Outcome and cause of death in mental disorders of old age; a long-term follow-up of functional and organic psychoses. Acta Psychiatr. Scand. 38, 249–276

Kay, D.W.K., Bergmann, K., Foster, E., Garside, R.F. (1966): A four year follow-up of a random sample of old people originally seen in their own homes. A physical, social, and psychiatric enquiry. Proc. 4th World Cong. Psychiatry, pt 3, pp. 1668–1670

Kay, D.W.K. (1972): Epidemiological aspects of organic brain disease in the aged. In: Aging and the Brain. Gaitz, C.M. (ed.). New York: Plenum Press, pp. 15–27

Kral, V.A. (1962): Senescent forgetfulness; benign and malignant. Can. Med. Assoc. J. 86, 257–260

Kral, V.A. (1967): Stress reactions in old age. Laval Med. 38, 561–566

Kral, V.A. (1973): Psychiatric problems in the aged: a reconsideration. Can. Med. Assoc. J. 108, 584–590

Klatzo, I., Gajdusek, D.C., Zigas, V. (1959): Pathology of Kuru. Lab. Invest. 8, 799–847

Klüver, H., Bucy, P.C. (1939): Preliminary analysis of functions of the temporal lobes in monkeys. Arch. Neurol. Psychiatry 42, 979–1000

Klüver, H. (1958): The "Temporal Lobe Syndrome" produced by bilateral ablations. In: Neurological Basis of Behavior. Woltensholme, G.E.W., O'Connor, M.E. (eds.). Boston: Little Brown, pp. 175–182

Krücke, W., Beck, E., Vitzthum, H.G. (1973): Creutzfeldt-Jakob disease. Some unusual morphological features reminiscent of Kuru. Z. Neurol. 206, 1–24

Larson, T., Sjogren, T., Jacobson, G. (1963): Senile dementia, a clinical, sociomedical, and genetic study. Acta Psychiatr. Scand. 39 (Suppl. 167), 1–257

Lauter, H., Meyer, J.E. (1968): Clinical and nosological concepts of senile dementia. In: Senile Dementia. Müller, C., Ciompi, L. (eds.). Bern: Huber, pp. 13–26

Lhermitté, J., Nicolas, M. (1924): La démence sénile et ses formes anatomo-cliniques. L'Encephale 19, 583–654

Libow, L.S. (1973): Pseudo-senility: acute and reversible organic brain syndromes. J. Am. Geriatr. Soc. 21, 112–120

Lorenzo, A.V., Bresnan, M.J., Barlow, C.F. (1974): Cerebrospinal fluid absorption deficit in normal pressure hydrocephalus. Arch. Neurol. 30, 387–393

Lowenberg, K., Rothschild, D. (1931): Alzheimer's disease. Its occurrence on the basis of a variety of etiological factors. Am. J. Psychiatry 11, 269–285

Maudsley, H. (1868): The Physiology and Pathology of Mind. London: MacMillan

McCarron, M.M., McCormick, R.A. (1965): Acute Organic Disorder Accompanied by Mental Symptoms. Calif. Dept. of Mental Hygiene

McHugh, P. (1964): Occult hydrocephalus. Q. J. Med. 33, 297–308

Mercier, C. (1905): Sanity and Insanity. London: Walter Scott

Messert, B., Baker, N.H. (1966): Syndrome or progressive spastic ataxia and apraxia associated with hydrocephalus. Neurology 16, 440–452

Messert, B., Wannamaker, B.B. (1974): Reappraisal of the adult occult hydrocephalus syndrome. Neurology 24, 224–231

Milhorat, T.H. (1972): Hydrocephalus and the Cerebrospinal Fluid. Baltimore: Williams and Williams

Moses, S.G., Robins, E. (1975): Regional distribution of norepinephrine and dopamine in brains of depressive suicides. Psychopharmacol. Bull. 1, 327–337

Nauta, W.J.H. (1962): Neural association of the amygdaloid complex in the monkey. Brain 85, 505–519

Nevin, S., McNenemey, W.H., Behrman, S., Jones, D.P. (1960): Subacute spongiform encephalopathy – a subacute form of encephalopathy attributable to vascular dysfunction (spongiform cerebral atrophy). Brain 83, 519–563

Ojemann, R.G., Fisher, C.M., Adams, R.D., Sweet, W.H., New, P.F.J. (1969): Further experience with the syndrome of "normal" pressure hydrocephalus. J. Neurosurg. 31, 279–294

Papez, J.W. (1937): A proposed mechanism of emotion. Arch. Neurol. Psychiatry 38, 725–743

Pearce, J. (1974): The extrapyramidal disorder of Alzheimer's disease. Eur. Neurol. 12, 94–103

Perry, E.K., Perry, R.H., Blessed, G., Tomlinson, B. (1977): Necropsy evidence of central cholinergic deficits in senile dementia. Lancet 1, 189

Pilleri, G. (1966): The Klüver-Bucy syndrome in man. A clinico-anatomical contribution to the function of the medial temporal lobe structures. Psychiatr. Neurol. Med. Psychol. 152, 65–103

Post, F. (1951): The outcome of mental breakdown in old age. Br. Med. J. 1, 436–440

Post, F. (1962): The significance of affective symptoms in old age. Maudsley Mono No. 10. London: Oxford University

Post, F. (1966): Somatic and psychic factors in the treatment of elderly psychiatric patients. J. Psychosom. Res. 10, 13–18

Post, F. (1968): The development and progress of senile dementia in relationship to the functional psychiatric idsorders of later life. In: Senile Dementia. Muller, C., Ciompi, L. (eds.). Bern: Huber, pp. 85–100

38

Reis, D.J. (1974): Consideration of some problems encountered in relating specific neurotransmitters to specific behaviors or disease. J. Psychiatr. Res. 11, 145–148

Roos, R., Gajdusek, D.C., Gibbs, C.J. (1973): The clinical characteristics of transmissible Creutzfeldt-Jakob disease. Brain 96, 1–20

Rose, F.C., Symonds, C.P. (1960): Persistent memory defect following encephalitis. Brain 83, 206–212

Roth, M. (1955): The natural history of mental disorder in old age. J. Ment. Sci. 101, 289–301

Roth, M., Tomlinson, B.E., Blessed, G. (1967): The relationship between quantitative measures of dementia and of degenerative changes in the cerebral grey matter of elderly subjects. Proc. R. Soc. Med. 60, 254–258

Roth, M., Myers, D.H. (1969): The diagnosis of dementia. Br. J. Hosp. Med. 2, 705–717

Rothschild, D. (1956): Senile psychoses and psychoses with cerebral arteriosclerosis. In: Mental Disorders in Later Life. Palo Alto: Stanford University Press, 2nd edition, pp. 289–331

Savage, G. (1920): Mental disorders associated with old age. J. Nerv. Ment. Dis. 51, 217–230

Scoville, W.B., Milner, B. (1957): Loss of recent memory after bilateral hippocampal lesions. J. Neurol. Neurosurg. Psychiatry 20, 11–21

Seidler, H., Malamud, N. (1963): Creutzfeldt-Jakob disease. Clinico pathologic report of 15 cases and review of the literature (with special reference to a related disorder designated as subacute spongiform encephalopathy). J. Neurophatol. Exp. Neurol. 22, 381–402

Shakespeare, W. (1947): The Tragedy of King Lear. Brooke, T., Phelps, W.L. (eds.). New Haven: Xale University Press

Shenkin, H.A., Greenberg, J., Bouzarth, W.F., Gutterman, P., Morsales, J.O. (1973): Ventricular shunting for relief of senile symptoms. J. Am. Med. Assoc. 225, 1486–1489

Shildkraut, J.J. (1965): The catecholamine hypothesis of affective disorders: a review of supporting evidence. Am. J. Psychiatry 122, 509–522

Shopsin, B., Wilk, S., Sathananthan, G., Gershon, S., Davis, K. (1974): Catecholamines and affective disorders revised: a critical assessment. J. Nerv. Ment. Dis. 158, 369–383

Sjögren, H. (1964): Paraphrenic melancholic and psychoneurotic states in the presenile-senile period of life. Acta Psychiatr. Scand. (Suppl.) 176, 1–64

Skae, D., Clouston, T.S. (1974): Morisonian lectures on insanity for 1873. J. Ment. Sci. 20, 1

Spillane, J.A., White, P., Goodhardt, M.J., Flack, R.H.A., Bowen, D.M., Davison, A.N. (1977): Selective vulnerability of neurons in organic dementia. Nature 226, 558–559

Sohn, R.S., Siegel, B.A., Gado, M., Torack, R.M. (1973): Alzheimer's disease with abnormal cerebrospinal fluid flow. Neurology 23, 1058–1065

Sourander, P., Sjögren, H. (1970): The concept of Alzheimer's disease and its clinical implications. In: Alzheimer's Disease and Related Conditions. Wolstenholme, G.E.W., O'Connor, M.E. (eds.). London: Churchill, pp. 11–32

Strecker, E.A., Ebaugh, F.G. (1951): Practical Clinical Psychiatry. Philadelphia: Blakiston, 7th edition

Strecker, E.P., James, A.E., Konigsmark, B., Merz, T. (1974): Autoradiographic observations in experimental communicating hydrocephalus. Neurology 24, 192–197

Taylor, James (1931): Selected Writings of John Hughlings Jackson. Basic Books, New York, 2, 13, 414–416

Terzian, H., Ore dalle, G. (1955): Syndrome of Klüver and Bucy reproduced in man by bilateral removal of the temporal lobes. Neurology 5, 373–380

Tomlinson, B.E., Blessed, G., Roth, M. (1970): Observations on the brains of demented old people. J. Neurol. Sci. 11, 205–242

Torack, R.M. (1975): The role of norepinephrine in the function of the area postreme III. Participation of nerve endings in altered uptake and release of tritiated norepinephrine. In: Brain-Endocrine Interaction II. Knigge, K.M., Scott, D.E., Kobayashi, H., Ishii, S. (eds.). Basel: Karger, pp. 204–216

Traub, R., Gajdusek, D.C., Gibbs, C.J., Jr. (1977): Transmissible virus dementia. In: Aging and Dementia. Smith, W.L., Kinsbourne, M. (eds.). Jamaica: Spectrum, pp. 91–172

Weller, R.O., Wisnieski, H. (1969): Histological and ultrastructural changes with experimental hydrocephalus in adult rabbits. Brain 92, 819–828

Wood, H.C. (1887): Nervous Diseases and their Disorders. Philadelphia: Lippincott

Worster-Drought, C., Greenfield, J.G., McNenemey, W.H. (1944): A form of familial dementia with spastic paralysis. Brain 67, 38–43

Yakovlev, P.I. (1948): Motility, behavior, and the brain. Stereodynamic organization and neural co-ordinates of behavior. J. Nerv. Ment. Dis. 107, 313–335

3. Diagnostic Tests of Dementia as Research Tools

In a real sense, the methodologies that have been used to diagnose brain disease consti-
tute research modalities and vice versa. Dementia is an exclusively human problem, so in
one way or another the research on dementia must involve the human brain. Human
experimentations is severely restricted, so ordinary animal procedure is not possible.
Therefore, the study of human brain disease by these diagnostic methods may be the
main source of information during the active phase of the dementing process. The major
problem in all these studies is the definition of normal, particularly when it becomes
identified with age. However, when valid criteria of normalcy are established these techniques afford us a great opportunity to investigate the pathogenetic mechanisms of
dementia. Unlike the autopsy, they can always be applied to evolving dementia so that
subtle deviations from the normal may be more apparent. The effectiveness with which
this is done becomes of interest not only to the diagnostician but also to all neurobio-
logists.

Psychological Tests of Intelligence

The psychological concept of intelligence has been expressed by Wechsler (1944) in the
following way:

> Intelligence is the aggregate or global capacity of the individual to act purposefully, to think
> rationally and to deal effectively with his environment.

This definition is of interest, since the mental abilities of thinking and purposeful
activity seem to be requisites for an effective confrontation between man and the world
he lives in. This definition appears to anticipate MacLean (1970), who states:

> All conventionally recognized forms of psychological information – awareness, sensations. per-
> ceptions, compulsions, affects, thoughts – are characterized by a co-existing state of subjectivity.

So the "motility of effectiveness" of Yakovlev (1948), the subjectivity of MacLean
(1970) and "the (ability) to deal effectively with his environment" (Wechsler, 1944)
become uniformly important considerations of the neocortical function we recognize as
intelligence. However, in virtue of its abstract and subjective nature this vital component
of intelligence is the least adaptable to measurement.

Early psychologists appear to be quite aware of this problem and it seems very reasonable that the more tangible aspects of intelligence, i.e., vocabulary, memory, language,
design should become the areas selected for formalized testing. Even these pursuits did
not appear to be successful until Spearman (1904) and Binet and Simon (1911) decided
to pool the results of different testing areas rather than to consider them as individual

indicators of intelligence. This multifactorial or composite concept of intelligence continued until Alexander (1935) determined that verbal and practical aspects of intelligence are separate and independent. His ideas became formalized in the verbal and performance scales of the Wechsler-Bellevue Intelligence Test (Wechsler, 1939) which evolved into the Wechsler Adult Intelligence Scale (WAIS) in 1955.

Throughout this period, the abstract and subjective aspects of intelligence were reflected by the inclusion of a "g" factor (Spearman, 1927) and the "X" and "Z" factors (Alexander, 1935). Even as late as 1943, Wechsler spoke of the importance of these subjective factors, which ironically became nonintellective:

> When our scales measure the non-intellective as well as the intellectual factors in intelligence, they will more nearly measure what in life corresponds to intelligent behavior.

After 1943, interest in these areas waned perceptibly.

The popularity of testing for practical and verbal intelligence appears to be the reason for the demise of subjectivity in psychometries. This enthusiasm arose from the fact that a differential development has been shown in children and an independent decay has been noted in adults. Practical (performance) intelligence increases until about age 15; it remains constant for a decade and then begins a progressive decline to death. Verbal intelligence, however, continues to develop at least until the 5th decade and even after 65 there is little deterioration in this area (Riegel, 1959). In this way the validity of these scales became established and they were accepted as indices of normal development and normal aging.

The deterioration of intellect with increasing age has been established since 1932 (Miles and Miles) and has been a most consistent and well-documented finding ever since (Fox and Birren, 1950; Botwinick, 1967). In this psychological conception of brain degeneration verbal scales remain intact (hold category) and performance declines (nonhold). The ultimate result of aging is dementia and Alzheimer's disease is premature aging, which is precisely what many clinical investigators have been saying for years:

> Psychiatrists and neurologists have been primarily concerned with the latter (dementia) and have almost entirely disregarded what, for want of a better term, we shall refer to as normal mental deterioration. Psychologically, however, there is little difference between the two, except as regards the rate at which deterioration occurs, and, in the case of traumatic injury, as regards the number of mental functions involved. The deterioration met with in normal old people is similar to that met with in most organic brain diseases. Senility, or extreme mental deterioration, is merely a terminal state of certain processes which begin relatively early in life and continue progressively with age. The net result of the accompanying changes is to impair all original endowment. Whether we wish to reserve the term mental deterioration to cover only the extreme losses of ability or pefer to apply it equally to the entire senescent decline is a matter of convenience. (Wechsler, 1944.)

As soon as the decay of practical intelligence had become well defined, there followed an application of the same tests to people with mental disease. Earlier studies such as that by Cameron (1938) reveal surprising conclusions:

> It is not without general significance that our senile group, in spite of devastating memory deficits and hopeless disorientation, in its use of the instruments of communication was definitely superior to our schizophrenics who knew where they were, who the experimenter was, what the year and season were and when and where they were born.

But by 1944 the Bellevue scale had been sophisticated and accepted as the assay technique. The report by Rabin in 1945 appeared to confirm the aging-related concept of dementia:

No significant differences in psychometric patterns between the several senile diagnostic groups of the patient population were obtained.

The discrepancies between verbal and performance scales, frequently considered as an indicator of inefficiency, tend to be largest in senile psychosis.

However, by 1951, Botwinick and Birren (1951a) had finished their own study of senile psychosis and could not duplicate the findings of Rabin:

The subtests which show the largest decline with age did not show the greatest differences in the two groups of this study. Thus the digit symbol subtests, which declines most with age, showed a smaller difference between the two groups than did the information subtests, which declines least with age. If deterioration in the senile psychoses were essentially a process of accelerated aging the subtests which show the largest age changes might be expected to show the largest differences between the two groups.

This distinction from normal aging was reported again by Dorken in 1954:

. . . it can be demonstrated by psychological tests that senile dementia is qualitatively as well as quantitatively different from normal senescent decline, is independent of it and probably superimposed on it,

and by Orme in 1957:

A decline with age of verbal performance seems to be important in the senile dementia group, distinguishing them from normals of approximately the same age range.

Finally in 1972, Overall and Gorham subjected their results of psychometrics in aging and dementia to multivariate statistical analysis and drew the following conclusion:

This is not to say that there may not be an organic basis for the poor performance of old persons, but the nature of the organic component is surely different from that in patients with clinical brain syndrome. We conclude that normally aging individuals are not marching along the road to chronic brain syndrome. Older persons tend to manifest selective performance deficits, but the pattern is distinct from the deficit that is evident in persons suffering clinical brain disease.

It is quite apparent that these tests of intelligence have refuted the theory that the decline of aging is a prelude to senile decompensation. However, in recent years several investigators (Eisdorfer et al., 1970; Botwinick, 1967) have shown that these tests are unfairly biased against the older adult. The time factor as well as social and motivational factors affect the elderly much differently than the young. Accordingly there are new efforts to design a test for old people (Botwinick and Storandt, 1973). It is quite possible that a new appreciation of adult intelligence will emerge at some future date. Until that time, the status of psychometric in aging is either that of an experimental procedure, or of a proof that aging and senile dementia are different.

Organic dementia has been shown to be prognostically distinct from functional psychoses, yet there is a definite symptomatic overlap with depression (Kiloh, 1961) and acute confusional states (Kral, 1973). For this reason, a very definitive benefit would accrue from an ability of psychometric testing to afford diagnostic and prognostic distinction between these perplexing clinical syndromes. Various attempts have been made to demonstrate diagnostic usefulness, but the results are very inconsistent. Even the separation of organic and functional disease has not been reported by everyone. Cameron (1938) believed that senile dements performed better than schizophrenics, while Rabin (1945) and Walton (1958) found lower levels for performance in senile psychotics. Neither Rabin or Walton could find qualitative differences in test patterns but Roth and Hopkins (1953) and Cowan et al. (1975) report that the two groups can be distinguished accurately. A difference between arteriosclerotic and senile psychosis would appear to be even more difficult and Botwinick and Birren (1950) could offer no basis for their separation. Yet Hopkins and Roth (1953) and Perez et al. (1975) believe this is possible. An accurate evaluation of these reports is practically impossible, since the subject material varies, the tests are not uniform, and there are only infrequent follow-up.

This lack of distinctive patterning would seem to preclude the use of psychometrics as a predictive index of senile mental disorder. Several investigators (Nott and Fleminger, 1975; Inglis et al., 1960; Walton, 1958) have arrived at this conclusion as a result of their retrospective studies. However Whitehead (1976), Folstein et al. (1975) and Blessed et al. (1968) do not agree and each of them has devised a test that is believed to be predictive of outcome. The interesting aspect of these tests is that only one (Whitehead, 1976) uses an established intelligence test and this is only one part of the evaluation. A major component of each is an evaluation of nonintellective factors such as awareness and effective behavior. The test devised by Blessed et al. (1968) is predictive not only of outcome, but also of the presence of senile plaques (SP) and neurofibrillary tangles (NF) in the brain. This is the best examples of psychometrics being predictive of brain damage.

The usefulness of traditional testing programs to reveal brain damage appears to be restricted chiefly by the lack of a test designed specifically for this purpose. Botwinick and Birren (1951) had very quickly noted this deficiency in the WAIS but it continues in use for the lack of a better substitute. Yates (1969) wrote of this dilemma most plaintively:

> It is doubtful whether any aspect of psychological testing has been more indadequately treated than the diagnostic assessment of brain damage.

Several aspects of this impasse appear worthy of comment. The first concerns the concept of "brain damage". This term has absolutely no meaning to a pathologist, to whom it is pure folly to include in one category meningioma, glioma, porencephaly, and cortical laceration among many others of equal diversity (McFie and Piercy, 1952). Actually the singular lack of pathologic correlation in these studies is so striking that even an understanding of abnormal brain volume is rarely possible. The second comment concerns the nature of these mental disorders in the aged. We have already noted that intellectual (cortical) dysfunction occurs in AD but that this is a relatively late and inconsistent aspect of the problem. Abnormal behavior may be prominent early and is inevitable terminally. It would seem to be significant that the only psychological study that has been shown to have pathologic predictability is the evaluation of competent behavior by Blessed et al. (1968). Furthermore Whitehead (1976) and Folstein et al. (1975) have shown that some combination of intellectual and nonintellective factors can have diagnostic and predictive value. Any new test of adult intelligence that does not include nonintellective factors would appear to have questionable significance for senile dementia. This seems to be an indication that this condition is not primarily neocortical dysfunction.

Electrocencephalography

A most perplexing aspect of the dementia enigma concerns the failure of the EEG to afford more insight into its nature and course. The EEG is a scientific, objective, reproducible measurement of neuronal electrical activity. A very reasonable assumption would be that some distinctive change would occur in this function incident to neuronal injury in dementing syndromes. Yet, with the exception of Creutzfeldt-Jakob disease (CJD), the modern electroencephalography (EEG) has little diagnostic or predictive importance for dementia. Such disappointment is commonplace in mental diesease but this one is particularly discouraging because the EEG has been the most sophisticated diagnostic tool during the last 40 years.

The EEG measures localized electrical activity at eight or more standardized areas of the scalp from electrodes that are believed to record activity chiefly from the underlying cortex. The tracing is believed to be the summation of the various potentials [membrane potentials, postsynaptic potentials (PSPs)] generated by nervous tissue. Currently a major contribution is believed to be derived from the numerous PSPs, both inhibitory and excitatory, generated in the cortex. The cellular components of the nervous system that are involved in these PSPs include the dendritic network from adjacent nerve cell bodies (Clare and Bishop, 1955), synaptic boutons of neurons chiefly located in other parts of the brain, and the local glial cell population.

According to this arrangement, the EEG could be affected by a distant injury, altering the synaptic input of an area, and by a local process changing glial cells or dendrites. The oligodendroglia are believed to regulate the ionic environment to prevent prolonged or exaggerated electrical responses (Ransom and Goldring, 1973). They may have a significant role in convulsive disorders (Ransom, 1974). However, specific oligodendroglial disease chiefly occurs in white matter (subacute sclerosing encephalitis, multiple sclerosis) and a reduction of synaptic input must be massive to become apparent (Chatrian et al., 1964). So the major determinant of the abnormal EEG is considered most often to be the local dendritic network.

For this reason, focal changes in the EEG have been interpreted generally to indicate local disease. This has been particularly useful in focal epilepsy where accurate localization of epileptiform foci is a prerequisite for surgical resection. Pathologic examination of resected temporal lobes has revealed that 72% had some anatomic counterpart (Cavanagh et al., 1958). For this reason electroencephalographers have developed and maintained a close correlation with pathology. These same attitudes have been applied to a study of diffuse disorders such as occur in dementia, especially since focal abnormalities can exist superimposed on a diffuse change. With ragard to dementia, this attitude becomes translated into a conviction that it is a brain disease, which is in marked contrast to the belief of most psychologists that it is essentially an aging process.

Early EEG studies of dementia have chiefly involved senile and arteriosclerotic psychosis (Hoch and Kubis, 1941; Liberson and Seguin, 1945). These studies reveal that a high incidence of abnormal slow activity is correlated with brain atrophy. This pattern is not considered an early change, since many of these dements do have normal EEGs and the abnormal tracings become more common as the disease progresses. No distinction is made between senile psychosis and arteriosclerotic psychosis. In addition, Greenblatt (1944) called attention to the fact that the EEG becomes abnormal in the aged and many of the changes seen in mental disorders are explicable on this basis.

Several investigators, most notably Obrist (1951) now began to be interested in the EEG changes of normal aging. These studies were eventually to demonstrate quite conclusively that slowing and spread of alpha activity is more common in the elderly (Mengoli, 1952; Obrist, 1953). Moreover, focal changes, particularly of theta and delta activity are noted to occur quite commonly in the temporal lobe (Busse and Obrist, 1963; Kooi et al., 1964). These changes in the EEG are not considered to be the result of normal aging but rather of an *age-related disorder,* particularly vascular disease. An important reason for this is that these changes are not present uniformly, so they cannot be considered an inevitable consequence of aging. The vascular origin of these focal changes is also suggested by their occurrence in people with some form of vascular problem (Obrist, 1963). An important aspect of these studies is that they involve mentally competent individuals so that the focal abnormalities especially are considered to have prognostic value as indicators of incipient vascular disease. Sheridan (1954) even considered that an abnormal EEG 3 weeks before a stroke could have been an indication of cerebral vascular insufficiency. Unfortunately no difference in survival rate could be demonstrated between two groups of elderly subjects with and without EEG changes, particlarly abnormal temporal lobe foci (Obrist, 1972; Busse and Obrist, 1963).

The more recent EEG studies of dementia seem to have been correctly designed: They include a control population, both functional and organic brain diesease, repetitive testing with clinical appraisal, and finally a remarkable degree of pathologic correlation (Muller and Kral, 1967; Mundy-Castle et al., 1953; Swain, 1959; Sheridan et al., 1955). Three changes in the EEG have been observed in these studies: (1) slow alpha rhythm, (2) focal or diffuse theta activity, (3) focal or diffuse delta activity. The following conclusions appear in these studies:

1. Abnormal EEGs occur more commonly over the age of 65 but all these patterns can occur in younger people, especially focal abnormality of the temporal lobe (Kooi et al., 1974).
2. Somewhat less than half (31%–46%) of senile dements will have a normal EEG (Mundy-Castle et al., 1953; Sheridan et al., 1954; Barnes et al., 1956).
3. The abnormal EEGs that occur in functional psychosyndromes can be explained on the basis of age (Barnes et al., 1956). An increased number of abnormal EEGs are found in organic psychoses but there is no characteristic pattern that can be used to distinghuish senile dementia and arteriosclerotic psychosis (Sheridan et al., 1954; Barnes et al., 1956; Liberson and Seguin, 1945).
4. Apart from CJD and in some cases of Huntington's chorea no distinctive EEG changes can be considered diagnostic of a form of dementia. A specific change of low-amplitude waves (Sishta, 1974) is seen in 30% of patients with Huntington's chorea. Frontal intermittent rhythmic delta slow activity has been considered a criterion for successful shunting of NPH. This has not been substantiated by other studies (Hughes, 1975) and the change is not specific for NPH.

Nevin has described the EEG changes of CJD in his characterization of subacute spongiform encephalopathy in 1960:

Three features are to be noted. 1) A partial or complete obliteration of the normal rhythms. 2) Widespread high voltage slow activity associated with generalized sharp wave complexes which are mainly monophasic or diphasic. 3) Periodic intermission of the slow and sharp wave activity by runs of lower voltage; slow activity, an intermission which may be conspicuous and regularly recurring or on the other hand little evident.

Later, the periodicity was emphasized by Burger et al. (1972) who noted increasing frequency to the point of being continuous. The latter was considered a grave prognostic sign.

The EEG changes in animals with transmissible viral dementia (TVD) have been described by Cathala et al. (1973). Changes in recordings from indwelling electrodes could be observed 8 months before the animal develops altered clinical behavior. At the onset of minor clinical changes, the EEG is described as being "generally slow and disorganized in marked contrast to the behavior of the animal". Polyphasic periodic activity becomes increasingly frequent after the 12th month and eventually becomes continuous. The EEG appears to have diagnostic and prognostic significance both in human CJD and in animal TVD.

While senile dementia frequently is accompanied by abnormal EEG, in the routine EEG there is at present no change that can be used to diagnose senile dementia. The incidence of abnormal records has been stated to increase in terminal dementia, suggesting that repetitive tracings might reveal a change. However, Sheridan et al. (1954) have repeated the EEG every 3 months for 2 years and have observed every type of variation including improvement. Perhaps a more encouraging aspect of this dilemma is the study of sensory evoked responses using photic stimulation. Kooi et al. (1957), Straumanis et al. (1965), Muller and Kral (1967), as well as Visser et al. (1976) have all noted polyphasic responses to slowly repeated stimuli which have not been observed in normal aged subjects or in functional mental disease. Pathologic study of 13 such patients (Muller and Kral, 1967) has revealed senile dementia and AD in 11 cases. The other brains also had distinct pathology, one having multiple infarcts while the other had Wernicke's encephalopathy.

Recently, another study of evoked responses has resulted in a new concept of brain dysfunction in senile dementia. Gerson et al. (1976) have used computer analysis to evaluate the responses of both hemispheres to both visual and auditory stimuli. Normally the responses are symmetrical, but in senile dementia they are asymmetrical. The authors suggest that dementia brain is less well coordinated than the brain of a normal aged person. If these results can be duplicated, a new role may be indicated for the EEG in dementia.

Pathologic correlation with abnormal EEG always has been a high priority but has been successful only in about half of the cases (Sheridan et al., 1954; Swain, J.M., 1959). Even in temporal lobe epilepsy nonspecific medial sclerosis or no change was seen in 36 of 50 brains (Cavanagh et al., 1958). The reason for such poor performance is due undoubtedly to the fact that there is no generally used reliable histologic technique that demonstrates dendrites, synapses, or oligodendroglia. Recent studies of slow virus encephalopathy (Lampert et al., 1975) have shown that dendritic changes are present. Synaptic involvement in aging rats (Bondareff and Geinisman, 1976) and in SP is well documented (Gonatas et al., 1967). The dendritic network can be demonstrated histologically using Golgi impregnation (Colon and Smit, 1970) and Aghajanian and Bloom (1967) have devised a useful technique to stain synapses. Any meaningful evaluation of the abnormalities in EEG recordings would seem to require an assay of underlying cortex using techniques as well as a quantitative determination of plaques and tangles.

Radiographic Technique

Radiographic techniques have become essential in the differential diagnosis of dementia but they have revealed no information relevant to the question of whether aging or disease cause dementia. The major reason for this impasse consists in the lack of information on normal aging that has been or can be obtained. No one has a pneumoencephalogram or an angiogram as part of an annual physical. Until the advent of computerized cranial tomography (CT) in 1973 all these diagnostic techniques were invasive and as such each had a distinct morbidity, which precluded their use on normal people. Oldendorf (1961) aptly deplores this situation:

> As a practicing clinical neurologist, I am daily confronted with the necessity of performing these traumatic tests (angiography and ventriculography), because the information obtained is so vital to intelligent case management. . . Each time I perform one of these primitive procedures, I wonder why no more pressing need is felt by the clinical neurological world to seek some technique which would yield direct information about the brain structure without traumatizing it.

Pneumoencephalography has been a major diagnostic technique in the evaluation of dementia particularly as a determinant of cortical atrophy and ventricular enlargement. However the procedure frequently causes temporary headache and, more important, an aggravation of dementia, especially in NPH. Therefore the method has its major value as a single diagnostic study and is not used repetitively as a research tool.

The use of radioactive labels has assumed its greatest value in cisternography as a study of CSF dynamics. As a determinant of reduced CSF flow it has become essential in the diagnosis of NPH. Degrees of ventricular reflux and location of blocks are readily demonstrable. These studies also revealed that a component of communicating hydrocephalus may be superimposed upon AD (Coblentz et al., 1972). The demonstration of some alteration of CSF dynamics is a sine qua non for any consideration of shunt therapy. These labels have also been used to study CSF-brain exchange at the ependymal level (Strecher et al., 1974) and absorption of CSF (Siegel, 1974). However there are no data applicable to a study of possible distinction between aging and disease as a mechanism for dementia. The use of labeled markers in measurements of cerebral blood flow will be considered later as part of the discussion of vascular diesease as a cause of dementia.

At present the radiographic technique that is most applicable for the study of the dementia problem appears to be CT. This noninvasive technique has no morbidity and there is no contraindication to repetitive testing other than the cost of the procedure. Furthermore it is the only radiographic technique capable of yielding direct information about the cellular character of the brain. In this regard pneumoencephalography is of least value, since it enables observations only of intracranial spaces and any concept of brain pathology must be deduced from some alteration of these spaces, i.e., brain atrophy is indicated by increased air overlying the cerebral convexities. Blood flow measurement and angiography reveal considerable insight into vascular dynamics but neurons are extravascular units and, while obviously dependent upon blood flow, they survive semiautonomously in the extravascular brain.

CT, in contrast to these previous techniques, purports to evaluate brain cells. Attenuation of the energy of an X-ray probe by passage through the cells of the brain is recognized and computed as a measure of tissue density (Hounsfield, 1973). Water is the standard by which the instrument is calibrated for a zero reading. By these standards fat and lipids have an attenuation value of -30. Heavy metals, especially iron and calcium, have a relevance to brain tissue and produce a logarithmic attenuation of the probe according to their concentration. In this way an image of the brain is constructed so that the ventricles, because of their fluid content, have very low density. White matter in virtue of its high lipid content is less dense than grey matter but significantly higher than the ventricles.

With a 160 x 160 matrix the instrument evaluates a mass of tissue 1.5 x 1.5 x 13 mm, so there is no question of evaluating cells other than collectively. Discrimination is also restricted by a fluctuation in the output of the energy of the X rays (Rutherford et al., 1975). When these problems are resolved efficient quantitative assay of small amounts of tissue will occur. Even with the present system variations from normal brain attenuation can be very accurately recognized in cerebral hematomas and in most brain tumors.

The importance of CT for dementia is twofold: (1) A normal aging population may be evaluated safely for the first time, and (2) repetitive evaluation of abnormal brain tissue is realistic. At this time it is impossible to predict what type of information will eventually emerge from these studies, especially when histologic and/or biochemical correlations are appreciated more completely. In the most thorough study to date (Torack et al., 1976) water and cell destruction were associated with reduction of attenuation values while blood, calcium, iron, and gliosis were present in elevated values.

Current CT studies of dementia are used chiefly to detect cerebral atrophy and ventricular enlargement. Diffuse or localized cortical atrophy and a characterization of ventricular outline can be demonstrated with an efficiency comparable to the pneumoencephalogram (Gawler et al., 1976; Huckman et al., 1975; Baker et al., 1974). The results of these studies have revealed a more precise relationship between normal ventricular and brain size (Synek et al., 1976). The normal width of hemispheral sulci has been measured by Gyldensted and Kosteljanitz (1976). The enlargement of the lateral ventricles during normal aging has been evaluated by Barron et al. (1976). When these baseline studies had been completed the application of CT to a study of senile dementia was considered to be feasible. Several interesting observations have been reported recently. Roberts and Caird (1976) have noted ventricular enlargement to correlate with a mental impairment that has been observed by psychometrics, but no significant degree of cortical atrophy has been found. In another study of dements, diffuse slowing on the EEG has been used as the marker of dementia and once again, no correlation with cerebral atrophy could made (Stefoski et al., 1976). I believe a very reasonable prediction is that a new appreciation of cerebral atrophy will result from CT studies, particularly those of the early stages of dementia and those which involve a 3 dimensional reconstruction of brain volume.

Morphologic and Chemical Assay of Brain Tissue

The opportunity to evaluate morbid anatomy at an autopsy has been the traditional source of ultiamte disease characterization. We have noted already how the major morphologic correlate of dementia, i.e., NF and SP, lack specificity, not only for dementing disease but also for a distinction from normal aging. Lacking a pathognomonic morphology, this brain tissue has been studied more recently by means of biochemical assays. The early studies (Pope et al., 1964; Suzuki et al., 1965; Cherayil, 1969) revealed

Table 3.1. Follow-up survey of dementia biopsy patients

	Patient	Age: onset	Clinical diagnosis	Biopsy diagnosis	Course	Autopsy diagnosis
1.	J.R.	53	Dementia 2 months	CJD	D, 1.5 months	CJD
2.	D.R.	74	Dementia 1 month	CJD	D, 2 months	No autopsy
3.	J.S.	36	Dementia 9 months	Enceph.	D, 6 months	No autopsy
4.	M.M.	58	NPH 2 years	Enceph.	A, 2 years	
5.	E.N.	69	NPH 2 months	AD	D, 3 months	No autopsy
6.	L.L.	57	Dementia 4 years	AD	D, 6 months	AD
7.	E.B.	58	Dementia 5 years, NPH	AD	D, 9 months	No autopsy
8.	E.P.	62	Dementia 2 years	AD	D, 6 months	No autopsy
9.	F.S.	53	Dementia 3 years	AD	A, 4 years	−
10.	R.M.	63	Dementia with myoclonus 1 year	AD	A, 2.5 years	−
11.	J.M.	54	Dementia 1.5 years	AD	Lost	−
12.	I.M.	68	Dementia 3 years	AD	Lost	−
13.	W.C.	60	Dementia 6 years	AD	Lost	−
14.	M.F.	61	Dementia 3 years	AD	Lost	−
15.	F.F.	70	NPH 1 year	Early AD	D, 1 week	AD/CA
16.	R.W.	76	Stroke	AD/CA	D, 1 day	AD/CA
17.	T.B.	68	NPH 2 months	Normal	D, 6 months	No autopsy
18.	M.G.	25	Dementia 1 year	Normal	D, 8 months	Neuroaxonal dystrophy
19.	B.R.	62	NPH 2.5 years	Normal	D, 2 months	Subacute dementia
20.	R.E.	62	Dementia 1 year, NPH	Normal	D, 2.5 years	Subacute arteriosclerotic encephalopathy
21.	W.M.	46	Huntington's chorea chorea 15 years	Normal	D, 2 years	Huntington's chorea
22.	A.R.	58	NPH 1.75 year	Normal	D, 1.5 month	NPH
23.	E.L.	48	Dementia 1 year	Normal	A, 5 years	−
24.	R.A.	44	Dementia 1 year	Normal	A, 3 years	−
25.	B.G.	50	Dementia 1 year	Normal	A, 4 years	−
26.	F.E.	47	Dementia 15 years	Normal	A, 9 years	−
27.	M.F.	48	Dementia 5 years	Normal	A, 5 years	−
28.	M.P.	61	Subdural 3 months	Normal	A. 9 months	−
29.	R.M.	63	NPH 6 months	Normal	A, 3 years	−

D, dead
A, alive
NPH, normal pressure hydrocephalus
AD, Alzheimer's disease
CJD, Creutzfeldt-Jakob disease
CA, Congophilic Angiopathy

differences in acetyl cholinesterase, ganglioside, and glycolipid content of dementia brain that were considered secondary to neuronal loss. Increased acid polysaccharides were believed to reflect amyloid deposition in SP. More recently the absence of a neuronal protein, neuronin S-6, has been noted by Bowen et al. (1973), Smith and Bowen (1976), and Nishimura et al. (1975). We do not know the significance of this finding; the specific function of this protein is not defined at present. A new protein was reported by Iqbal et al. (1974) which has been considered to represent the abnormal NF. The chemistry of NF will be discussed in Chapter 6.

The fundamental defect in the use of autopsy material for these studies is that the autolytic changes incident to death quickly disrupt fine-structural detail and chemical properties, especially enzymatic activity. Therefore the other source of brain tissue, cerebral biopsy, has beem emphasized in recent years as being a much more suitable substrate for such investigation. Indeed the characterizations of NF (Terry, 1963), of SP (Terry et al., 1964), and of the biochemical components by Suzuki et al. (1965) have been a result of multivariate evaluation of cerebral biopsies. The major problems of biopsy study are the small size of the tissue sample and the lack of effective control material. Even with the abundant tissue available at autopsy, the quantitative distinction between the NF and SP content of normal and demented brains (Tomlinson et al., 1970) is extremely tedious and tenuous. In biopsy, the small amount of tissue available for assay precludes such detailed study. The difficulty of control can only be resolved by a comparison of biopsy and autopsy assay. This becomes a problem when these assay do not agree, as with the high glycolipids reported from biopsies by Suzuki et al. (1965) but not observed by Cherayil (1969) using autopsy material. The current role of brain biopsy in dementia diagnosis and research is being re-evaluated because of these difficulties.

The primary diagnostic objective of biopsy in dementia has been to establish the presence of AD. In this way Sim et al. (1966) and Smith et al. (1966) report the clinical and pathologic findings in a series of 56 biopsies, 35 of which were positive for AD. The major problems of biopsy diagnosis are illustrated in these reports: (1) why did 17 patients with clinically manifest dementia have a normal biopsy? (2) Did the normal occurrence of plaques and tangles in the elderly cause a false positive diagnosis of AD in the nine patients aged 60–69? Unfortunately these questions have never been resolved.

A personal experience with a variety of dementia has been gained during the past 10 years. A series of 29 biopsies has been studied using both light- and electron microscopy. Some cases were also investigated by means of histochemical methods demonstrating enzyme activity. The noteworthy aspects of these studies have been published previously (Torack, 1966. 1969, 1971; Torack and Hughes, 1972; Hughes et al., 1973). Several different morphologic and chemical peculiarities have been derived from these studies; however no etiologic relationships have been noted except in one case which has been considered to be compatible with a protein metabolic defect (Torack, 1966). A similar neuronal structural change was recently described in a case of Huntington's chorea (Tellez Nagel et al., 1973) and biochemical assay of this tissue has suggested a defect in histone metabolism (Iqbal et al., 1974a).

A clinical follow-up survey of these biopsied patients has been completed in order to afford additional insight into the prognostic value of a brain biopsy. The total number of biopsies is listed in Table 3.1 and only four cases have been completely lost to follow-up. The survival data are presented in Table 3.2. The diagnosis of CJD, as expected, has

Table 3.2. Average survival rate in dementia biopsy

Diagnosis	Dead	Alive
CJD (2)	3.3 months	
Encephalitis (1)	1.3 years	
(1)		4.0 years
AD (1)	5 months	
(3)	4.3 years	
(2)		5.2 years
AD/CA (2)	6 months	
Normal (3)	1.8	
(3)	6.9	
(7)		7.4 years

the worst prognosis, the two patients (# 1 and # 2) dying in 3.5 and 3.0 months respectively. Two cases of congophilic angiopathy (# 15 and # 16) also demonstrate a poor outcome with an average survival of 6 months. This is quite distinct from ordinary AD in which average survival to death is 4.3 years (# 6–8), and which also includes two patients (# 9, 10) alive after 7 and 3.5 years. Thirteen normal biopsies fall into two rather distinct groups. Three patients (# 17–19) had a subacute course and at least one of these (19) is considered to represent the nonspongiform variant of CJD (Hughes et al., 1972). Most important is the survival of patients with a normal biopsy. This group includes three people (# 20–22) who had an average clinical course of 6.9 years to death and seven patients (# 23–29) who are alive after a mean duration of 7.4 years. Only one case (# 5), a 69-year-old female, appears to have been misdiagnosed as AD because of age-related NF and SP.

Another very important aspect of this biopsy study is the benefit afforded by a subsequent autopsy. This dual assay permits an understanding of evolution unattainable in a single study, particularly when the time interval is reasonably short (less than a year). The most impressive change occurred in patient FF (# 15). This 70-year-old white male developed a slowly progressive dementia with leg weakness. After a year, a RISA cisternogram revealed ventricular reflux and impaired CSF flow compatible with NPH. A biopsy, obtained at the time of a shunt procedure, revealed foci of neuritic plaque formation and there were also some thickened blood vessels. A week later the patient died from massive intracranial hemorrhage. The cerebral cortex adjacent to the biopsy site (and in all other lobes), contained numerous well-formed plaques, many of them perivascular in location. Moreover the blood vessels had obvious congophilia with green birefringence in polarized light indicative of amyloid deposition. Electron microscopy confirmed the presence of amyloid in these blood vessels even in the biopsy. This rapid evolution of SP and vascular amyloidosis has not been even suggested in other autopsy studies (Torack, 1975).

In two other cases there was a remarkable association between a normal biopsy and an abnormal autopsy.

Case Report: M. G. (# 18) had a rapidly evolving dementing syndrome for a year when a diagnostic brain biopsy was performed. This biopsy was normal but she continued on her rapid course and died 8 months later. An autopsy evaluation revealed neuroaxonal dystrophy involving central white matter, corpus callosum, and corticospinal tracts. The cortex near the biopsy site revealed an extensive loss of neurons in the lower half of the cortex. This is a case of subcortical dementia and very deftly demonstrates the late evolution of neuronal destruction in comparison to the onset of dementia (Torack, 1972).

Case Report: R. E. (# 20) developed progressive dementia with a gait disturbance. The onset of a flu-like syndrome was accompanied by rapid deterioration with a left hemiparesis. A biopsy at that time was read as normal. Becuase of dilated ventricles and a cisternogram compatible with NPH, he was later shunted. Episodic worsening continued with an evolution of seizures and he expired 2.5 years after the biopsy. The autopsy revealed multiple foci of subcortical softening with demyelination in the central white matter. The cortex adjacent to the biopsy site revealed only mild diffuse neuronal loss and the process was considered compatible with subcortical sclerosis (Olszewski, 1962).

In summary, these two cases of dementia had a normal biopsy and they would not have been explained without the autopsy. Both were associated with subcortical pathology but the effect upon the cortex was quite different.

The primary justification of brain biopsy in dementia continues to derive from its diagnostic value as indicator of AD or CJD. However, combined morphologic and chemical assay, clinical follow-up, and subsequent autopsy examination greatly expand the information obtainable from a biopsy. Two unemphasized aspects of biopsy study deserve special consideration. First, the presence of normal tissue can have significant value not only as an indicator of potentially reversible disease but also as a prognosticator of prolonged survival. Secondly, repetitive study of brain tissue at biopsy may be the most effective procedure to reveal pathogenesis of dementia, particularly when the interval is short. It seems amazing that, at this time, no sequential assay of this type has been reported despite the number of brain biopsies performed yearly.

References

Aghajanian, G.K., Bloom, F.E. (1967): The formation of synaptic junctions in developing rat brain. A quantitative electron microscopic study. Brain Res. 6, 716–727

Alexander, W.P. (1935): Intelligence, concrete and abstract. Br. J. Psychol. Monograph.

Baker, H.L., Campbell, J.K., Houser, D.W., Reese, D.F., Sheedy, P.K., Holman, C.B. (1974): Computer assisted tomography of the head. An early evaluation. Mayo Clin. Proc. 49, 17–27

Barnes, R.H., Busse, E.W., Friedman, E.L. (1956): The psychological functioning of aged individuals with normal and abnormal electroencephalograms II. A study of hospitalized individuals. J. Nerv. Ment. Dis. 124, 585–593

Barron, S.A., Jacobs, L., Kinkel, W.R. (1976): Changes in size of normal lateral ventricles during aging by computerized tomography. Neurology 26, 1011–1013

Binet, A., Simon, T. (1911): A method of measuring the development of the intelligence of young children. Translated by C.T. Town. Lincoln/Ill.: Courier

Blessed, G., Tomlinson, B.E., Roth, M. (1968): The association between quantitative measures of dementia and of senile change in the cerebral grey matter of elderly subjects. Br. J. Psychiatry 114, 797–811

Botwinick, J., Birren, J.E. (1951a): The measurement of intellectual decline in the senile psychoses. J. Consult. Clin. Psychol. 15, 145–150

Botwinick, J., Birren, J.E. (1951b): Differential decline in the Wechsler-Bellevue subtests in the senile psychoses. J. Gerontol. 6, 365–368

Botwinick, J. (1967): Cognitive Processes in Maturity and Old Age. Berlin–Heidelberg–New York: Springer

Botwinick, J., Storandt, M. (1973): Speed functions, vocabulary, ability, and age. Precep. Mot. Skills 36, 1123–1128

Bondareff, W., Geinisman, Y. (1976): Loss of synapses in the dentate gyrus of the senescent rat. Am. J. Anat. 145, 129–136

Bowen, D.M., Smith, C.B., Davison, A.M. (1973): Molecular changes in senile dementia. Brain 96, 849–856

Burger, L.J., Rowan, J., Goldensohn, E.S. (1972): Creutzfeld-Jakob Disease. An electroencephalographic study. Arch. Neurol. 26, 428–433

Busse, E.W., Obrist, W.D. (1963): Significance of focal electroencephalographic changes in the elderly. Postgrad. Med. 34, 179–182

Cameron, N. (1938): A study of thinking in senile deterioration and schizophrenic disorganization. Am. J. Psychol. 51, 650–664

Cathala, F., Court, L., Rohmer, F., Gajdusek, D.C., Gibbs, C.J., Jr., Castaigne, P. (1973): Experimental transmission of Creutzfeldt-Jakob disease to a chimpanzee, with an electroencephalographic study using indwelling electrodes. Proc. X Int. Cong. Neurol., Int. Cong. Series No. 319, pp. 381–389

Cavanagh, J.B., Falconer, M.A., Meyer, A. (1958): Some pathogenic problems of temporal lobe epilepsy. In: Temporal Lobe Epilepsy. Baldwin, M., Bailey, P. (eds). Springfield: C.C. Thomas, pp. 140–148

Chatrian, G.E., Shaw, C.M., Liffman, H. (1964): The significance of periodic lateralized epileptiform discharges in EEG. An electrographic, clinical and pathological study. Electroencephal. Clin. Neurophysiol. 17, 177–193

Cherayil, G.D. (1969): Estimation of glycolipids in four selected lobes of human brain in neurological diseases. J. Neurochem. 16, 913–920

Clare, M.A., Bishop, G.H. (1955): Properties of dendrites: Apical dendrites of the cat cortex. Electroecephal. Clin. Neurophysiol. 7, 85–97

Coblentz, J.M., Maltis, S., Zingesser, L.H., Kasoff, E.S., Wisniewski, H.M., Katzman, R. (1973): Presenile dementia. Arch. Neurol. 29, 299–308

Colon, E.J., Smit, G.J. (1970): Quantitative analysis of the cerebral cortex II. A method for analyzing basal dendritic plexuses. Brain Res. 22, 363–380

Cowan, D., Wright, P.M., Gourlay, A.J., Smith, A., Barron, G., de Gruchy, J.R.M., Kelleher, M.J., Kellett, J.M. (1975): A comparative psychometric assessment of psychogeriatric and geriatric patients. Br. J. Psychiatry 127, 33–41

Dorken, H. (1954): Psychometric differences between senile dementia and normal senescent decline. Can. J. Psychol. 8, 187–194

Eisdorfer, C., Nowlin, J., Wilkie, F. (1970): Improvement of learning in the aged by modification of autonomic nervous system activity. Science 170, 1327–1329

Folstein, M.F., Folstein, S.E., McHugh, P.R. (1975): Mini-mental state. A practical method for grading the cognitive state of patients for the clinician. J. Psychiatr. Res. 12, 189–198

Fox, C., Birren, J.E. (1950): The differential decline of subtest scores of the Wechsler-Bellevue intelligence scale in 60–69 year old individuals. J. Genet. Psychol. 77, 313–317

Gawler, J., DuBoulay, G.H., Bull, J.W.D., Marshall, J. (1976): Computerized tomography (the EMI scanner): a comparison with pneumoencephalography and ventriculography. J. Neurol. Neurosurg. Psychiatry 39, 203–211

Gerson, I.M., John, E.R., Bartlett, F., Koenig, V. (1976): Average evoked response (AER) in the electroencephalographic diagnosis of the normally aging brain: A practical application. Electroencephal. Clin. Neurophysiol. 7, 77–91

Gonatas, N.K., Anderson, W., Evangelista, I. (1967): The contribution of altered synapses in the senile plaque. J. Neuropathol. Exp. Neurol. 29, 463–478

Greenblatt, M. (1944): Age and electroencephalographic abonormality in neuropsychiatric patients. Am. J. Psychiatry 101, 82–90

Gyldensted, C., Kosteljanetz, M. (1975): Measurements of the normal hemispheric sulci with computer tomography: A preliminary study on 44 adults. Neuroradiology 10, 147–149

Hoch, P., Kubis, J. (1941): Electroecephalographic studies in organic psychosis. Am. J. Psychiatry 98, 404–408

Hopkins, B., Roth, M. (1953): Psychological test performance in patients over sixty. II. Paraphrenia, arteriosclerotic psychosis and acute confusion. J. Ment. Sci. 99, 451–463

Hounsfield, G.N. (1973): Computerized transverse axial scanning (tomography): Part 1, description of system. Br. J. Radiol. 46, 1016–1022

Huckman, M.S., Fox, J., Topel, J. (1975): The validity of criteria for the evaluation of cerebral atrophy by computed tomography. Radiology 116, 85–92

Hughes, C.P., Myers, F.K., Smith, K., Torack, R.M. (1973): Nosologic problems in dementia. A clinical and pathologic study of 11 cases. Neurlogy 23, 344–351

Hughes, C.P. (1975): Personal communication

Iqbal, K., Wisnewski, H.M., Shelanski, M.L., Brostaff, S., Lewnicz, B.H., Terry, R.D. (1974): Protein changes in senile dementia. Brain Res. 77, 337–343

Iqbal, K., Tellez-Nagel, I., Grundke-Iqbal, I. (1974a): Protein abnormalities in Huntington's Chorea. Brain Res. 76, 178–184

Kiloh, L.G. (1961): Pseudo dementia. Acta Psychiatr. Scand. 37, 336–351

Kooi, K.A., Eckman, H.G., Thomas, M.H. (1957): Observations on the response to photic stimulation in organic cerebral dysfunction. Electroencephal. Clin. Neurophysiol. 9, 239–250

Kooi, K.A., Guvener, A.M., Tupper, C.J., Bagehi, B.K. (1964): Electroencephalic patterns of the temporal region in normal adults. Neurology 14, 1029–1035

Kral, V.A. (1973): Psychiatric problems in the aged: a reconsideration. Can. Med. Assoc, J. 108, 584–59

Lampert, P.W., Gajdusek, D.C., Gibbs, C.J., Jr. (1975): Pathology of dendrites in subacute spongiform virus encephalopathies. Adv. Neurol. 12, 465–470

Liberson, W.T., Seguin, C.A. (1945): Brain waves and clinical features in arteriosclerotic and senile mental patients. Psychosom. Med. 7, 30–35

MacLean, P. (1970): The triune brain, emotion and scientific bias. In: Neurosciences, Second Study Program. Schmitt, F.O. (ed.). New York: Rockefeller Univ., pp. 336–348

McFie, A., Piercy, M.F. (1952): Intellectual impairment with localized cerebral lesions. Brain 75, 292–311

Mengoli, G. (1952): The EEG in old age. Electroencephal. Clin. Neurophysiol. 4, 232–233

Miles, C.C., Miles, W.R. (1932): The correlation of intelligence scores and chronological age from early to late maturity. Am. J. Psychol. 44, 44–78

Muller, H.F., Kral, V.A. (1967): The electroencephalogram in advanced senile dementia. J. Am. Geriatr. Soc. 15, 415–426

Mundy-Castle, A.C., Hurst, L.A., Beerstecher, D.M., Prinsloo, T. (1953): The electroencephalogram in the senile psychoses. Electroencephal. Clin. Neurophysiol. 6, 245–252

Nevin, S., McNenemey, W.H., Behrman, S., Jones, D.P. (1960): Subacute spongiform encephalopathy – A subacute form of encephalopathy attributable to vascular dysfunction. (Spongiform cerebral atrophy). Brain 83, 556–563

Nishimura, T., Hariguchi, S., Tada, K., Kaneko, Z. (1975): Changes in brain water soluble proteins in presenile and senile dementia. In: Proc. VIIth Int. Cong. Neuropathol. Korney, St., Tariska, St., Gosztonyi, G. (eds.). Amsterdam: Excerpta Medica, Vol. 2, pp. 139–142

Obrist, W.D. (1951): The electroencephalogram of normal male subjects over age 75. J. Gerontol. Suppl. to No. 3, 2nd Ant. Geriat. Cong., September, pp. 130

Obrist, W.D. (1953): The electroencephalogram of normal aged adults. Electroencephal. Clin. Neurophysiol. 6, 235–244

Obrist, W.D. (1963): The electroencephalogram of healthy aged males. In: Human Aging: A Biological and Behavioral Study. Birren, J.E., et al. (eds.). Bethesda/Md.: U.S. Gov't Printing Off.

Obrist, W.D. (1972): EEG and intellectual function in the aged. Electroencephal. Clin. Neurophysiol. 33, 253

Oldendorf, W.H. (1961): Isolated flying spot detection of radiodensity discontinuities displaying the internal structure of a complex object. IRE Trans. Biomed. Econ. 8, 68–72

Olszewski, J. (1962): Subcortical arteriosclerotic encephalopathy. World Neurol. 3, 359–375

Orme, J.E. (1957): Non verbal and verbal performance in normal old age, senile dementia and elderly depression. J. Gerontol. 12, 408–413

Overall, J.E., Gorham (1972): Organicity versus old age in objective and projective test performance. J. Consult. Clin. Psychol. 39, 98–105

Perez, F., Rivera, V.M., Meyer, J.S., Gay, J.R.A., Taylor, R.L., Mathew, N.T. (1975): Analysis of intellectual and cognitive performance in patients with multi-infarct dementia, vertebrobasilar insufficiency with dementia, and Alzheimer's disease. J. Neurol. Neurosurg. Psychiatry 38, 533–540

54

Pope, A., Hess, H.H., Lewin, E. (1964): Studies on the microchemical pathology of human cortex. In: Morphological and Biochemical Correlates of Neural Activity. Cohen, M.M., Snider, R.S. (eds). New York: Hoeber, pp. 98–111

Rabin, A. (1945): Psychometric trends in senility and psychoses of the senium. J. Gen. Psychol. 32, 149–162

Ransom, B., Goldring, S. (1973): Slow depolarization in cells presumed to be glia in cerebral cortex of cat. J. Neurophysiol. 36, 869–878

Ransom, B. (1974): The behavior of presumed glial cells during seizure discharge in cat cerebral cortex. Brain Res. 69, 83–99

Riegel, K. (1959): A study of verbal achievements of older persons. J. Gerontol. 14, 453–456

Roberts, M.A., Caird, F.I. (1976): Computerized tomography and intellectual impairment in the elderly. J. Neurol. Neurosurg. Psychiatry 39, 986–989

Roth, M., Hopkins, B. (1953): Psychological test performance in patients over sixty. I. Senile psychosis and the affective disorders of old age. J. Ment. Sci. 99, 439–450

Rutherford, R.A., Pullan, B., Isherwood, I., Goddard, J. (1975): Quantitative aspects of computer assisted tomography. Br. J. Radiol. 48, 605

Sheridan, F.P., Yeager, C.L., Oliver, W.A., Simon, A. (1955): Electroencephalography as a diagnostic and prognostic aid in studying the senescent individual. A preliminary report. J. Gerontol. 10, 53–59

Siegel, B.A., Johnson, E.W. (1974): Mesurement of intrathecal I^{131}-albumin transport to plasma. Neurology 24, 501–503

Sim, M., Turner, E., Smith, W.T. (1966): Cerebral biopsy in the investigation of presenile dementia. I. Clinical aspects. Br. J. Psychiatry 112, 127–133

Sishta, S.K., Troupe, A., Marszalek, K.S., Kremer, L.M. (1974): Huntington's Chorea: An electroencephalographic and psychometric study. Electroencephal. Clin. Neurophysiol. 36, 387–393

Smith, C.B., Bowen, D.M. (1976): Soluble proteins in normal and diseased human brain. J. Neurochem. 27, 1521–1528

Smith, W.T., Turner, E., Sim, M. (1966): Cerebral biopsy in the investigation of presenile dementia. II. Pathological aspects. Br. J. Psychiatry 112, 127–133

Spearman, C. (1904): General intelligence: Objectively determined and measured. Am. J. Psychol. 15, 202–285

Spearman, C. (1927): The Abilities of Man. New York: MacMillan

Stefoski, D., Bergen, D., Fox, J., Morrell, F., Huckman, M., Ramsey, R. (1976): Correlation between diffuse EEG abnormalities and cerebral atrophy in senile dementia. J. Neurol. Neurosurg. Psychiatry 39, 751–755

Straumanis, J.J., Shagass, C., Schwartz, M. (1965): Visually evoked cerebral response changes associated with chronic brain syndromes and aging. J. Gerontol. 20, 498–506

Strecker, E.P., James, E., Jr., Kelley, J.E.T., Merz, T. (1974): Semiquantitative studies of transependymal albumin movements in communicating hydrocephalus. Radiology 111, 341–346

Suzuki, K., Katzman, R., Korey, S.R. (1965): Chemical studies on Alzheimer's disease. J. Neuropathol. Exp. Neurol. 24, 211–224

Swain, J.M. (1959): Electroencephalographic abnormalities in presenile atrophy. Neurology 9, 722–727

Synek, V., Reuben, J.R., DuBoulay, G.H. (1976): Comparing Evans' index and computerized axial tomography in assessing relationship of ventricular size to brain size. Neurology 26, 231–233

Tellez-Nagel, I., Johnson, A.B., Terry, R.D. (1973): Ultrastructural and histochemical study of cerebral biopsies in Huntington's Chorea. Adv. Neurol. 1, 387–398

Terry, R.D. (1963): The fine structure of neurofibrillary tangles in Alzheimer's disease. J. Neuropathol. Exp. Neurol. 22, 629–642

Terry, R.D., Gonatas, N.K., Weiss, M. (1964): Ultrastructural studies in Alzheimer's presenile dementia. Am. J. Pathol. 44, 269–297

Tomlinson, B.E., Blessed, Roth, M. (1970): Observations on the brains of demented old people. J. Neurol. Sci. 11, 205–242

Torack, R.M. (1966): Ultrastructural and histochemical studies in a case of progressive dementia and its relationship to protein metabolism. Am. J. Pathol. 49, 77–97

Torack, R.M. (1969): Ultrastructural and histochemical studies of cortical biopsies in subacute dementia. Acta Neuropathol. 13, 43–55

Torack, R.M. (1971): Studies in the pathology od dementia. In: Dementia, the Failing Brain. Wells, C. (ed.). Philadelphia: F.A. Davis

Torack, R.M. (1972): Case Report: Neuroaxonal dystrophy in a case of subacute dementia. Acta Neuropathol. 22, 264–268

Torack, R.M. (1975): Congophilic angiopathy complicated by surgery and massive hemorrhage. Am. J. Pathol. 81, 349–366

Torack, R.M., Alcala, H., Gado, M., Burton, R. (1976): Correlative assay of computerized cranial tomography (CCT), water content and specific gravity in normal and pathological post mortem brain. J. Neuropath. Exp. Neurol. 35, 385–392

Visser, S.L., Stam, F.C., Van Tilburg, W., OpDen Velde, W., Blom, J.L., DeRijke (1976): Visual evoked response in senile and presenile dementia. Electroencephal. Clin. Neurophysiol. 40, 385–392

Walton, D. (1958): The diagnostic and predictive accuracy of the Wechsler memory scale in psychiatric patients over 65. J. Ment. Sci. 104, 1111–1118

Wechsler, D. (1939): The Measurement of Adult Intelligence. 1st edition, Baltimore: Williams and Wilkins

Wechsler, D. (1943): Non-intellective factors in general intelligence. J. Abnorm. Psychol. 38, 101–103

Wechsler, D. (1944): Measurement of Adult Intelligence. Baltimore: Williams and Wilkins

Wechsler, D. (1955): Manual for the Wechsler Adult Intelligence Scale. New York: Psychological Corp.

Whitehead, A. (1976): The prediction of outcome in elderly psychiatric patients. Psychol. Med. 6, 469–479

Yakovlev, P.I. (1948): Motility, behavior and the brain. Stereodynamic organization and neural coordinates of behavior. J. Nerv. Ment. Dis. 107, 313–335

Yates, A.J. (1969): The validity of some psychological tests of brain damage. In: Neuropsychological Testing in Organic Brain Dysfunction. Smith, W.L., Phillipus, M.J. (eds.). Springfield: C.C. Thomas, pp. 49–79

4. Treatment of Senile Dementia

A most amazing aspect of therapeutic considerations of dementia is the similarity of experiences occurring 75 years ago to those of modern medicine. For example, the usefulness of general supportive care is evident in the observations of Clouston (1884):

> Excitement and new things or ways or places or persons should be avoided. Old people take best with what they have been accustomed to.
>
> The diet is also very important. I find the first food of life to be the best at the opposite end of life. There is nothing like milk, given warm and in small quantities at a time, and often. Fatten your patient and you will improve him in mind.

Similar advice is given in 1900 by Berkley:

> Good food, good nursing and hygienic surroundings are essential. Many of the senile dements have to be cared for at their homes, and unless they are unmanageable and degraded in their habits this can be done, provided a capable and attentive nurse can be obtained.

The management of elderly dementia was recently reviewed by Arie (1973) who concluded:

> Old people with failing brains have these main needs: For security, because their capacity to function far outstrips their capacity for change: For stimulation because dementia especially when restricted mobility and sensory privation in the form of deafness of blindness are added to it, makes the world a frightening and lonely place, and for patience, because old people are slow, but time and again will astonish one by their capacity to "get there in the end".

The other aspect of treatment concerns actual medical management, and frustration was very evident very long ago:

> It is surprising in some cases how much improvement in the arterial condition may be accomplished by the use of suitable diet and drugs and how completely such measures fail with others. (Berkley, 1900.)

The history of drug therapy is replete with reports of initial success, which eventually are followed by observations of failure. The following remarks of Alexander (1972) appear appropriate:

> Unfortunately, this area (medical management) perhaps more than most others is strewn with methodological pitfalls; controls are difficult to implement and objective criteria of improvement are difficult to define, particularly since there is an almost complete lack of valid and reliable psychological measures suitable for longitudinal analysis of change. It is evident that before these or other methods of therapy can be properly evaluated, efforts must be made to establish what are optimum treatment conditions, what are the best treatment schedules, how long can changes be expected to last and which are the most suitable patients for different treatments.

A current appraisal of medical management reveals no effective treatment of Alzheimers's disease (AD), but various aspects of therapy do afford some insight into the nature of the disease. From this viewpoint, a review of these experiences appears necessary.

Acute Confusion

Earlier (Sect. 2) we have reviewed the concept of acute confusion, its similarity to early dementia, and its evolution in some cases into a chronic brain syndrome indistinguishable from AD. The important aspects of acute confusion are that it is not due to endogenous brain disease, that a wide variety of exogenous factors can cause it (Libow, 1973), and that it is reversible in at least 50% of all cases. Among the etiologic factors, drugs appear prominently, especially psychoactive agents, which alter transmitter dynamics either cholinergically (Snyder, 1975) or aminergically (Lavin and Alexander, 1975; Thornton, 1976). There is an increased susceptibility for drug-induced toxic dilirium in the elderly (Bergmann, 1974) and especially in senile dements (Prien et al., 1975). The alteration is not uniform, for although greater responses are evoked by depressant drugs, stimulant activity appears to be suppressed. The known effects of these drugs on various aspects of synaptic function suggests that some change is occurring at this site perhaps in the character of receptor foci. The interesting paradox is that drugs that are used to treat dementia can also cause it.

Circulatory Agents

The persistent belief that AD is due to vascular insufficiency has led to a popularity of any technique that could improve the presumed cerebral ischemia. Vasodilation (Stern, 1970; Goldberg and Shuman, 1966), anticoagulation (Walsh and Walsh, 1972), and hyperbaric oxygen (Thompson et al., 1976) are all designed for this purpose. All of these treatments are followed by a lack of any consistent benefit for dementia (Prien, 1973), which is to be expected, since the vascular basis of organic brain syndrome is limited to multi-infarct dementia. The hyperbaric oxygen story is of interest because it illustrates a sequence of events that are characteristic of dementia treatment. In 1969, Jacobs et al. had reported improved cognition in chronic brain syndrome following 15 days' exposure to two 90-min intervals of 100% oxygen at 2.5 atm. These findings were confirmed by several therapists (Boyle, 1974; Edwards and Hart, 1974), but denied by Goldfarb et al. (1972). In order to resolve this controversy, Thompson et al. (1976) conducted a thorough study of this procedure using psychological tests, EEG, and cerebral blood flow assay as objective criteria of brain function. No distinct change in any of these parameters was noted in 8 patients with cerebrovascular diesease or in 13 patients with moderate to severe dementia.

There is an interesting exception in the clinical effects of the vasoactive dihydrogenated ergot alkaloids (DEA) (Hydergine), which have been postulated to reduce cerebrovascular resistance (Geraud et al., 1963). Improved cognition and effective behavior was reported by several investigators of "cerebrovascular insufficiency" in the elderly (Gerin, 1969; Triboletti and Ferri, 1969). More recently a clinical comparison with papaverine, in confused elderly patients, prompted Rosen (1975) to conclude that the effects of DEA were not due solely to a hemodynamic effect. Actually, extensive study of the metabolic effects of DEA (Meier-Ruge et al., 1975) has revealed (1) inhibition of catecholamine reuptake, (2) normalization of catecholamine or sympathetic-stimulated Na^+/K^+-ATPase, Mg^{2+}-ATPase, and cAMP-adenylcyclase, (3) inhibition of brain-specific low Km-cAMP-PEase. They believe that these effects alter synaptic transmission and that any occurring vascular effects are secondary. It seems that a serious study of DEA in diagnosed AD is indicated.

Metabolic Stimulants

The concept that the aging brain is metabolically inefficient derives chiefly from the decreased memory and performance plus the increased reaction time demonstrable in intellectual testing. A variety of stimulant drugs have been used in order to reverse this decline, including analeptics such as Metrazol and sympathomimetics such as amphetamines. Although they have been observed to increase awareness and perhaps memory function, their side-effects on other brain or cardiac function seems to preclude their usefulness in AD (Hollister, 1975).

A more specific form of metabolic stimulation has evolved from the hypothesis that RNA is the molecular substrate for information processing (Hyden, 1960). In this way, defective memory is recent because insufficient RNA is being made to handle new information. Support for this idea is afforded by an increase in RNA in rats following learning (Hyden and Egyhazi, 1962) and by the improvement in human memory after RNA treatment (Cameron, 1958). The direct therapeutic effect has been disproved by the inability of RNA to cross the blood-brain barrier (Eist and Seal, 1965) or to stimulate protein synthesis after intracerebral injection (Sved, 1965). Instead, the mental improvement has been considered to be an effect of hyperuricemia, which occurs particularly after IV injection of RNA. In 1967, Kral et al. noted no improvement of memory after RNA treatment and no difference of serum uric acid between senescence and dementia. About the same time, magnesium pemoline had been used to stimulate RNA synthesis in rat neurons (Glasky and Simon, 1966). Eisdorfer et al. (1968) used pemoline to treat 13 patients with a mild to moderately severe chronic brain syndrome and found no difference in cognition or behavior from a group of matched controls. At the present time, there is no indication that these attempts to stimulate protein and more specifically RNA synthesis are of benefit for dementia.

In 1956, the usefulness of procaine in deferring aging was announced and, since that time, a continuing debate has surrounded its use and effectiveness (Aslan, 1974). Its myriad benefits included a 79.7% inprovement in "central nervous system degeneration" and 90.1% improvement of cerebrovascular disorders. Some chemical basis for a CNS effect has been supplied by the recognition that procaine plus benzoic acid (Gerovital-H_3) has mild monoamine oxidase inhibitory action (Yau, 1974). This effect seemed to explain its usefulness in elderly depression (Sakalis et al., 1974; Cohen and Ditman, 1974). But Kral et al. (1962) reported no change in senile or arteriosclerotic brain disease and Cohen and Ditman (1974) observed the poorest responses in severe depression and "organic brain syndrome". If Gerovital-H_3 has any ability to defer aging, its uselessness in senile dementia demonstrates the latter is not synonymous with aging.

Psychoactive Drug Therapy

The occurrence of functional mental syndromes in patients with organic brain disease suggests that they are another clinical aspect of the disordered brain. Earlier, in Section 2, we noted that affective disorders have been etiologically linked with vascular dementia, while schizophrenia was associated with senile psychosis. This affiliation implies that the structural changes of organic dementia are related to a physiologic abnormality that is similar to purely functional diesease. In both cases, the underlying problem is considered to be transmitter control. The similarity of clinical syndromes suggests that the character of the response to psychoactive drugs is also indistinguishable.

In the early stage of dementia this seems to be true, for several authors have commented on the therapeutic responses of psychosyndromes in dementia (Bergmann, 1974; Prien, 1973). Furthermore, several evaluations of drug effectiveness have been carried out in affective disorders of mixed etiology and no distinction has been made between functional and organic diesease (Goldstein, 1974; Hader et al., 1966; Chesrow et al., 1962). On the other hand, drug effectiveness in functional schizophrenia is not correlated with similar success in organic dementia (Hamilton and Bennett, 1962; Rada and Kellner, 1976). This discrepancy could be due to a greater disability of the organic subjects as suggested by Salzman and Shader (1975) or it could indicate some different mechanism for schizophrenia.

In the later phase of dementia, this situation is not present. Salzman and Shader are quite definite about this change:

A seeming contradiction of the law of initial values can be observed when the research population under consideration is primarily composed of patients with relatively unchanging chronic organic brain deterioration. As a group, these patients tend to show very little change, if any, on most of the usual affective, behavioral, cognitive, or perceptual measures employed in psychopharmacology research. Although these patients are the sickest, and most impaired of the geriatric population, they show the least change. If a drug is to be tested on this population, there is relatively little possibility for change, unless, of course, the drug is very powerful. In general, if a drug has a modest, yet potentially useful, therapeutic effect, research using chronically impaired geriatric subjects is not likely to demonstrate these effects.

The responsiveness of affective syndromes to drugs that are known to alter the chemical control of neural transmission is the basis for the concept that these conditions are the result of transmitter imbalance, especially of catecholamines (Schildkraut, 1965). Drug therapy purports to restore equilibrium through a variety of effects mainly involving the synaptic site. The evolution of unresponsiveness in organic dementia suggests that sufficient damage has occurred at that site to negate compensation by psychoactive drugs. In other words, transmitter imbalance has been replaced by transmitter collapse. In this sense, the affective disorder and the therapeutic response should be considered an essential component of AD.

Antiviral Therapy

In 1971, Braham selected amantidine as a therapeutic agent in Creutzfeldt-Jakob disease (CJD) because of its antiviral action and because it was known to cross the blood-brain barrier. He noted a dramatic clinical improvement of behavior and, perhaps more impressive, a return of an abnormal EEG to near normal. Sanders and Dunn (1973) reported two cases of CJD that were treated with amantidine. The first made a considerable initial improvement, which was sustained for 2 months, at which time he rapidly deteriorated and died. The brain was remarkable in that it did not have status spongiosis. The second case also had a remarkable improvement in clinical status and in EEG, which was sustained for 30 months, up to the time of the report. A last case report (Ratcliffe et al., 1975) recorded no improvement with amantidine and postmortem examination of the brain revealed spongiform encephalopathy. Certainly, these few cases do not permit conclusions about amantidine treatment. The dramatic nature of these responses, especially the EEG changes, render further clinical trial necessary in AD as well as in CJD.

Surgical Management

Shunt Therapy

The rationale for a diversion of CSF from ventricles to the blood is based upon the premise that obstructed flow of CSF results in an alteration of brain-CSF equilibrium impairing the function of periventricular brain. In some cases of normal pressure hydrocephalus (NPH), a dramatic reversal of a dementing syndrome can follow the installation of such a shunt (Hakim and Adams, 1965). Unfortunately, this clinical improvement is not predictable, even when rigid criteria for the diagnosis of NPH are established (Messert and Wannamaker, 1974). A very likely explanation is that improvement will occur only when the mechanism of compensation by the brain for the obstructed flow has not been completed.

The possibility that an element of CSF obstruction exists in AD is suggested by the presence of meningeal fibrosis and ventricular dilatation. Indeed, some cases have been recognized to have altered CSF dynamics during life, and AD cases at autopsy (Coblentz et al., 1973; Sohn et al., 1973). Accordingly, shunt therapy has been attempted in patients with brain atrophy, but there has been minimal evidence that the course of the dementia has been altered (Coblentz et al., 1973). Therefore, the presence of dilated ventricles in AD is still considered to occur as a secondary event to brain atrophy.

Carotid Surgery

There seems to be little doubt that carotid endarterectomy is a valuable treatment when cerebral ischemia is associated with occlusive disease of the carotid artery (Perry et al., 1975; Engell et al., 1972). There is also no question that organic dementia can occur as a result of multiple strokes, so it is quite possible that an occasional patient with multi-infarct dementia can be helped by carotid endarterectomy. Although Fisher (1951) linked senile dementia with carotid thrombosis, the latter is not considered to have causative significance. This precludes the use of endarterectomy to treat senile dementia.

Conclusions

The value of psychoactive drugs is well recognized as treatment of psychosyndromes early in dementia. Many of these drugs are also known to cause a dementing syndrome. The latter stages of AD have been characterized by unresponsiveness to drug therapy, which seems to indicate that transmitter failure has superseded imbalance. The changing pattern of drug effectiveness should mean that these psychosyndromes are an integral component of AD and not an emotional reaction to the organic problem. It also suggests that dementing syndromes are disorders of transmission caused by disease of the peripheral neuron.

All attempts to treat AD by improving brain circulation appear ineffective. Only DEA is considered to be of value and this seems to accrue from its transmitter effect, rather than from vasodilation. This is consistent with the concept that vascular disease is not a cause of AD. Similar lack of success follows the use of metabolic stimulants, which implies that AD is more than slowing down (mental aging). Gerovital-H_3 has been considered to stimulate anabolic cellular processes and to defer aging, but no effect on senile dementia has been demonstrated. Surgical management is restricted to NPH and to a rare case of multi-infarct dementia. Perhaps, the only glimmer of hope lies in the amazing response to amantidine by three patients with CJD, but genuine enthusiasm must await further clinical trial.

References

Alexander, D.A. (1972): "Senile Dementia": A changing perspective. Br. J. Psychiatry 121, 207–214

Arie, T. (1973): Dementia in the elderly; management. Br. Med. J. 4, 602–604

Aslan, A. (1974): Theoretical and practical aspects of chemotherapeutic techniques in the retardation of the aging process. In: Theoretical Aspects of Aging. Rockstein, M. (ed.). New York: Academic Press, pp. 145–156

Bender, A.D. (1965): A pharmacodynamic basis for changes in drug activity associated with aging in the adult. Exp. Gerontol. 1, 237–247

Bergmann, K. (1974): Assessment of therapy in psychogeriatric illness. Gerontol. Clin. 16, 54–63

Berkley, H.J. (1900): A Treatise on Mental Disease. Appleton, New York

Boyle, E., Aparicio, A., Canosa, F., Owen, D., Dash, H.H. (1974): Hyperbaric oxygen and acetazolamide in the treatment of senile cognitive functions. Fifth Int. Hyperbaric Conf. 1, 432–438

Braham, J. (1971): Jakob-Creutzfeldt disease: Treatment by Amantidine. Br. Med. J. 4, 212–213

Cameron, D.E. (1958): The use of nucleic acid in aged patients with memory impairment. Am. J. Psychiatry 114, 943

Chesrow, E.J., Kaplitz, S.E., Breme, J.T., Musci, J., Sabatini, R. (1962): Use of new benzodiazepine derivative (Valium) in chronically ill and disturbed elderly patients. J. Am. Geriatr. Soc. 10, 667–670

Clouston, T.S. (1884): Clinical Lectures on Mental Disease. Philadelphia: Leas and Son

Coblentz, J.M., Mattis, S., Zengesser, L.H., Kasoff, S.S., Wisnieswki, H.M., Katzman, R. (1973): Presenile dementia: Clinical aspects and evaluation of cerebral-spinal fluid dynamics. Arch. Neurol. 29, 299–308

Cohen, S., Ditman, K.S. (1974): Gerovital-H_3 in the treatment of the depressed aging patient. Psychomatics 15, 15

Edwards, A.E., Hart, G.M. (1974): Hyperbaric oxygenation and the cognitive functioning of the aged. J. Am. Geriatr. Soc. 22, 376–379

Eisdorfer, C., Conner, J.F., Wilkie, F.L. (1968): The effect of magnesium pemoline on cognition and behaviour. J. Gerontol. 23, 283–288

62

Eist, H., Seal, U.S. (1965): The permeability of the blood-brain barrier (BBB) and blood cerebrospinal fluid barrier (BLB) to C^{14} tagged ribonucleic acid (RNA). Am. J. Psychiatry 122, 584–586

Engell, H.C., Boysen, G., Ladegaard-Petersen, H.J., Henriksen, H. (1972): Cerebral blood flow before and after carotid endarterectomy. Vasc. Surg. 6, 14–19

Fisher, C.M. (1951): Senile dementia – a new explanation of its causation. Can. Med. Assoc. J. 65, 1–7

Geraud, J., Bess, A., Rascal, A., Delpla, M., Marc-Vergnes (1963): Measurement of cerebral blood flow using Krypton 85. Some physiopathological and clinical applications. Rev. Neurol. 108, 542–557

Gerin, J. (1969): Symptomatic treatment of cerebrovascular insufficiency with Hydergine. Curr. Ther. Res. 11, 539–546

Glasky, A.J., Simon, L.N. (1966): Magnesium pemoline: Enhancement of brain RNA polymerases. Science 151, 702–703

Goldberg, R.I., Shuman, F.I. (1966): Pentamethylene-tetrazol, vasodilator, vitamin therapy for mentally confused geriatric patients: Double blind study. J. Am. Geriatr. Soc. 12, 589–593

Goldfarb, A.I., Hochstadt, N.J., Jacobson, J.H., Weinstein, E.A. (1972): Hyperbaric oxygen treatment of organic mental syndrome in aged persons. J. Gerontol. 27, 212–217

Goldstein, S.E. (1974): The use of mesoridazine in geriatrics. Curr. Ther. Res. 16, 316–323

Hader, M., Schulman, P.M., Madonick, M.J. (1966): Paranoid conditions of late life treated with Trifluoperazine. Dis. Nerv. Syste. 27, 460–462

Hakim, S., Adams, R.D. (1965): The special clinical problem of symptomatic hydrocephalus with normal cerebrospinal fluid pressure. J. Neurol. Sci. 2, 307–327

Hamilton, L.D., Bennett, J.L. (1962): The use of Trifluoperazine in geriatric patients with chronic brain syndrome. J. Am. Geriatr. Soc. 10, 140–147

Hollister, L.E. (1975): Drugs for mental disorders of old age. J. Am. Med. Assoc. 234, 195–198

Hyden, H. (1960): The neuron. In: The Cell: Biochemistry, Physiology, Morphology. Brachet, J., Mirsky, A.E. (eds.). New York: Academic Press

Hyden, H., Egyhazi, E (1962): Nuclear RNA changes of nerve cells during a learning experiment in rats. Proc. Natl. Acad. Sci. 48, 1366–1372

Jacobs, E.A., Winter, P.M., Alvis, H.J., Small, S.M. (1969): Hyperoxygenation effect on cognitive functioning in the aged. N. Engl. J. Med. 28, 753–757

Kral, V.A., Solyom, L., Enesco, H.E. (1967): Effect of short-term oral RNA therapy on the serum uric acid level and memory function in senile versus senescent subjects. J. Am. Geriatr. Soc. 15, 364–372 .

Kral, V.A., Cahn, C., Deutsch, M., Mueller, H., Solyom, L. (1962): Procaine (Novocain) treatment of patients with senile and arteriosclerotic brain disease. Can. Med. Assoc, J. 87, 1109–1113

Lavin, P., Alexander, C.P. (1975): Dementia associated with Clonidine therapy. Br. Med. J. 1, 628

Libow, L.S. (1973): Pseudo-senility: Acute and reversible organic brain syndrome. J. Am. Geriatr. Soc. 21, 112–120

Meier-Ruge, W., Enz, A., Gygax, P., Hunziker, O., Iwangoff, P., Reichlmeier, K. (1975): Experimental pathology in basic research of the aging brain. In: Aging, Volume 2. Gershon, S., Raskin, A. (eds.). New York: Raven Press, pp. 55–126

Messert, B., Wannamaker, B.B. (1974): Reappraisal of the adult occult hydrocephalus syndrome. Neurology 24, 224–231

Perry, P.M., Drinkwater, J.E., Taylor, G.W. (1975): Cerebral function before and after carotid endarterectomy. Br. Med. J. 4, 215–216

Prien, R.F., Haber, P.A., Coffey, E.M. (1975): The use of psychoactive drugs in elderly patients with psychiatric disorders: Survey conducted in twelve Veteran Administration hospitals. J. Am. Geriatr. Soc. 23, 104–112

Prien, R.F. (1973): Chemotherapy in chronic organic brain syndrome – A review of the literature. Psychopharmacol. Bull. 9, 5–20

Rada, R.T., Kellner, R. (1976): The effects of Thiothixene in geriatric patients with chronic brain syndrome. Psychopharmacol. Bull. 12, 30–32

Ratcliffe, J., Rittman, A., Wolf, S., Verity, M.A. (1975): Creutzfeldt-Jakob disease with focal onset unsuccessfully treated with Amantidine. Bull. Los Angeles Neurol. Soc. 40, 18–20

Rosen, H.J. (1975): Mental decline in the elderly: Pharmacotherapy (Ergot alkaloids versus Papa-verine). J. Am. Geriatr. Soc. 23, 169–174

Sakalis, G., Oh, D., Gershon, S., Shapsin, B. (1974): A trial of Gerovital-H$_3$ in depression during senility. Curr. Ther. Res. 16, 59–63

Salzman, C., Shader, R.I. (1974): Psychopharmacology in the aged. Research considerations in geriatric psychopharmacology. J. Geriatr. Psychoatry 7, 165–184

Sanders, W.L., Dunn, T.L. (1973): Creutzfeldt-Jakob disease treated with Amantidine. J. Neurol. Neurosurg. Psychiatry 86, 581–584

Shildkraut, J.J. (1965): The catecholamine hypothesis of affective disorders: A review of supporting evidence. Am. J. Psychiatry 122, 509–522

Snyder, B.D. (1975): Physostigmine. Antidote for anticholinergic poisoning. Minn. Med. 58, 456–477

Sohn, R.S., Siegel, B.A., Gado, M., Torack, R.M. (1973): Alzheimer's disease with abnormal cerebro-spinal fluid flow. Neurology 23, 1058–1065

Stern, F.H. (1970): Management of chronic brain syndrome secondary to cerebral arteriosclerosis with special reference to papaverine hydrochloride. J. Am. Geriatr. Soc. 18, 507–512

Sved, S. (1965): The metabolism of exogenous ribonucleic acid injected into mice. Can. J. Biochem. 43, 949–958

Thompson, L.W., Davis, G.C., Obrist, W.D., Heyman, A. (1976): Effects of hyperbaric oxygen on behavioral and psychological measures in elderly demented patients. J. Gerontol. 31, 23–28

Thornton, W.E. (1976): Dementia induced by methyldopa with haloperidol. N. Engl. J. Med. 294, 1222

Triboletti, F., Ferri, H. (1969): Hydergine for treatment of symptoms of cerebrovascular insuffi-ciency. Curr. Ther. Res. 11, 609–620

Walsh, A.C., Walsh, B.H. (1972): Senile and presenile dementia: Further observations on the benefits of a dicumarol-psychotherapy regimen. J. Am. Geriatr. Soc. 20, 127–131

Yau, T.M. (1974): Gerovital-H$_3$, monoamine oxidases and brain monamines. In: Theory of Aging. Rockstein, M. (Ed.). New York: Academic Press, pp. 157–165

5. Epidemiology of Dementia

General Considerations

The validity of dementia epidemiology as an etiologic determinant can be questioned on the basis of statistical accuracy and because the topic is redundant. The subjectivity of mental disorder is so great that most objective criteria of mensuration are not effective as a source of meaningful data. We have noted this failure in psychometrics, EEG, and pathologic studies. The usefulness of statistics to amplify causal relationships of insanity was briskly treated by Bell in 1844:

> No reason has presented itself to justify receding from the views presented for several years past, of the unsoundness and consequent uselessness of what are called the *statistics* of insanity. Every year's experience convinces me that those facts regarding this subject, which are capable of being arithmetically noted, are of too little moment to be worth recording at all, while those circumstances touching the duration, form, symptoms and event of cases, which would be truly important are, from their nature, incapable of being generalized tabularly into even a loose approximation to the truth. Statistics are doubtless valuable in relation to topics where accuracy is capable of being approached, but not in a legitimate mode of expressing mere opinions.
>
> I still find it impracticable in a vast proportion of cases, to fix with any certainty the point at which the mind lost its balance, and by which the duration of disease before admission can be determined, notwithstanding the great body of our inmates are from the intelligent and educated classes of society, where facts of this sort are attainable, if at all. I still find insanity rarely produced from a single cause, so marked as to permit being tabularized accurately, but by a combination or accidental coincidence of causes, moral, physical and educational.

The question of redundancy arises from the very concept of senile dementia. The name derives from mental decay with age and increasing susceptibility with prolonged life has always been accepted. The epidemiology of this deterioration was set forth by a pathologist, Warthin, in 1928:

> While there are great individual variations, these functions (intellectual and spiritual life) of the central nervous system usually are preserved in physiologic old age and may increase in value until about the 65th year when some impairment of memory and mental reaction may begin to show; after 70 the retrogression of cerebral function proceeds rapidly so that in those who reach or pass the 80th year a characteristic picture of "second childhood" develops.

About the only problem with this generalization has concerned the "great individual variations". Women have been considered more susceptible than men but this has never been well defined. Note the curious evaluation of women by Blandford in 1878:

> . . . Ladies frequently do not take care of themselves or their affairs at any time of their lives, nor do they pretend or claim to do so. Many could not who are yet of sound mind and able to make a will. You must take this into account when you are examining ladies with a view to testing their mental strength or weakness.

Curiously the writers of the 19th century do not seem to be impressed with any relationship between intelligence and dementia but this concept has been espoused more
recently by Vernon (1947):

> Our data tend to support, though they do not allow us to prove, the hypothesis of differential
> decline. If confirmed, it is of the greatest psychological and educational importance, since it suggests
> that men who make the most use of their intelligence retain it best, and that men in unskilled and
> laboring occupations tend to lose the mental capacities they possessed when they left school.

Finally Bevan Lewis (1899) considers the role of environment:

> . . . There is a most powerful agency in operation in a large number of such cases in the surround-
> ing conditions of life. Undue cerebral excitation, whether in the form of excessive mental work, and
> especially when prolonged intellectual operations are associated with anxiety and worry . . . such
> agencies operate for all (especially) at an age when the brain cells have reached their limit of normal
> functional activity . . . in the downward retrogressive changes of senility.

These opinions semm to indicate a multifactorial basis for senile dementia yet until
the last 25 years most statistical studies of dementia have involved only hospitalized
patients in mental institutions. Accurate concepts of prevalence, heredity, geographic
distribution, and even sex predilection were not possible until these surveys included the
population at large. An important factor in the evolution of such work was the general
acceptance of Roth's classification of mental disease in the elderly (1955). Apart from
making these studies correlative, functional syndromes were distinguished from organic
disease, and senile dementia could be separated from arteriosclerotic psychosis, so the
epidemiology of senile dementia per se became possible. As we begin an evaluation of
these studies, a more modern and positive approach to epidemiology than the cynicism
of Bell would appear laudable. The view of Austin and Werner (1974) seems refreshing:

> Epidemiology is the study of how and why diseases are distributed in the population the way
> they are . . . in other words, the study of why some get sick and some don't. Epidemiologists consider
> epidemiology to be a science. Actually, epidemiology is just a way of looking at things in a slightly
> different way . . . because you appreciate what things are important.

Previous Surveys of Senile Dementia

Cross-Sectional Survey

The first comprehensive survey of the prevalence of dementing syndromes in a general
population was that of Essen-Moller in 1956. He found that 5.5% of a rural Swedish
population had mild or serious dementia. This was a higher figure than that of earlier,
more limited studies but was corroborated by a prevalence of 4.8% in survey by Gruenberg (1959) in New York State. Since that time, numerous investigators have studied
the problem in various countries including Japan, Iceland, Norway, England, and Denmark. Five of these surveys have been selected for review in order to illustrate the data
derived from these efforts.

1. Kay et al. (1964). This is a survey of the 65+ population estimated to be 9031 in
five different electoral wards of an English industrial city. The mental symptoms were
noted to be mild or severe according to the criteria of Roth (1955). These people were
identified by home interview of 297 residents and by investigation of 208 institution-

alized citizens. The home interviews took place during a 4-month period which was succeeded by a follow-up interview 12–18 months later. The institutionalized cases were part of the hospital census of a single day.

2. Bollerup (1975). This is a study of 626 persons aged 70, all of whom lived in nine Copenhagen suburbs on census day May 1, 1967. Among these people, 588 were interviewed over a subsequent 18-month period, and information about another 38 was considered valid. Diagnostic criteria appear to be those of Roth.

3. Akesson (1969). The population includes that of two rural islands off the coast of Sweden. The occurrence of mental disease in persons aged 60+ was determined by a survey of institutionalized patients. Domiciliary cases were identified by means of some informant. The survey occurred during a 3-year period. The patients were diagnosed according to the criteria of Roth (1955).

4. Hagnell (1970). This is a 10-year follow-up of the survey by Essen-Moller in mainland rural Sweden. Originally 2550 persons comprised the area of study of which 443 were 60+ and interviewed by Essen-Moller. Hagnell evaluated 244 persons 60+ 10 years later, and used the same criteria for diagnosis as Essen-Moller (Roth, 1955).

5. Nielsen (1962). A study of the 65+ population of Samso island in Denmark, which is a relatively affluent rural society. These people could be identified because they are registered in the family care program. Nine hundred ninety-four probands were identified and formed 16.1% of the total population. The prevalence of dementia was completed during a 6-month period in 1961. Senile dementia and arteriosclerotic dementia were assayed using the criteria of Roth (1955).

These surveys have certain similarities. They appear to involve uniform criteria for diagnosis. They all involve both institutionalized and domiciliary persons within a fairly close geographic area (England, Sweden, Denmark). Obvious differences include the restriction to a single age group (Bolerup), the comparison of urban (Kay et al., Bollerup) with rural populations (Hagnell, Nielsen, Akesson). Finally there are distinct variations in the collection of the data so that no two surveys are exactly alike.

The data obtained in these surveys are presented with regard to prevalence (Table 5.1), sex (Table 5.2), and age (Table 5.3). The disparity in the prevalence of senile dementia illustrates the difficulty in comparing studies of this type. Bollerup's restrictive age criteria are unique. Akesson's low estimate may be related to the inclusion of persons 60–64, to the diagnostic criterion of constant confusion, or to the effectiveness of his contacts in identifying domiciliary cases. Another problem is the method of reporting the data, for only Hagnell reports his data as average annual incidence during a 10-year interval. With such discrepancies of methodology, it is difficult to establish etiologic distinction. However, when prevalence is as different as 0.38% and 18.2%, a massive difference between urban and rural population is suggested and needs varification. One conclusion that may be derived from these studies is that a constant relationship between disease rate, people, and environment has not been proven.

Similar problems arise in the consideration of sex and age. The sex distribution of senile dementia is predominately female according to Kay et al. and Akesson, but Hagnell, Bollerup, and Nielsen find it to be more common among males. A male predominance is more clearly demonstrated in arteriosclerotic psychosis. The occurrence of senile dementia according to age is similarly confused by a lack of comparable data. Kay et al. do not even offer an age breakdown of their cases. The most serious defect in most of these studies is that there is no complete age breakdown of the elderly population. The oldest members are usually lumped as 75+ or 80+. Without more complete age distribution any consideration of age relationships appears premature.

Table 5.1. Prevalence of dementia (percentage of proband population) in cross-sectional survey

Author	Age Group	Number of probands	SD	AS	Other	Total
Kay et al. (1964)	65+	505	4.2	3.9	1.9	10.0
Bollerup (1975)	70	626	1.3	2.0	1.9	5.2
Akesson (1969)	60+	4198	0.38	0.52		0.9
Hagnell (1970)	60+	443	16.1	3.6		19.7
Nielsen (1962)	65+	994	18.2	2.8		21.0

SD, senile dementia; AS, arteriosclerotic dementia

Table 5.2. Sex occurrence of dementia (percentage of proband population) in cross-sectional surveys

Author	SD		AS		Other	
	M	F	M	F	M	F
Kay et al. (1964) [a]	2.6	5.2	8.7	1.0	0.9	2.6
Bollerup (1975)	1.2	0	1.4	0.5	1.3	0.5
Akesson (1969)	0.12	0.26	0.26	0.26		
Hagnell (1970)	8.4	7.7	2.7	0.9		
Nielsen (1962)	10.2	8.0				

SD, senile dementia; AS, arteriosclerotic dementia; M, male; F, female.
a This includes only the probands living in the community.

Table 5.3. Age characteristics of dementia in cross-sectional survey (percent incidence)

Author	60–64	65–69	70–74	75–79	80–84	85–89	90+
Kay et al. (1964)							
Bollerup (1975)			5.0				
Akesson (1969)	0.1		0.43		0.36		
Hagnell (1970)	4.7		7.7		3.6		
Nielsen (1962)	—	1.6	3.4	4.7	5.0	3.4	

Larsson Survey

The one major survey that has included a complete breakdown of age (in 5-year intervals) is the study of senile dementia by Larsson et al. (1963). In contrast to the community surveys just described, the Larsson survey is a retrospective (case control) study of senile dementia in Stockholm, Sweden. The proband cases were selected from hospitalized patients who were accepted only after re-examination by one of the investigators. The diagnostic criteria were those of Roth.

The selection of these cases was not entirely random. Since a primary objective was to study a genetic influence on dementia, comparable numbers of male and female cases were selected. In this way 347 males and 372 females comprised this group, yet Larsson et al. Noted that only 24% of the patients in these mental hospitals were male. In addition only persons born within Sweden were included. The age (onset) distribution of the 719 cases is shown in Table 5.4. A representation of age distribution as a percentage of the Stockholm population revealed an increasing risk occurrence up to the 85–89 age group. A further increase was not noted after 90.

Table 5.4. Distribution by age of senile dementia in Stockholm according to the survey of Larsson et al. (1963)

Age group	60–64	65–69	70–74	75–79	80–84	85–90	90+
Probands	20	54	82	94	50	20	5
Stockholm population 1960	44,435	36,445	27,740	17,786	9,070	3,085	790
Morbidity risk [a]	0.045	0.1	0.29	0.53	0.55	0.65	0.64

[a] The morbidity risk is computed as a percentage of the Stockholm population for 1960 in each age group

Autopsy Studies

Another major difficulty of all clinical surveys is the 25% error in the distinction of mental disorder in the aged. This was noted quite definitely by Corsellis (1962):

Whenever a given type of change was expected in a particular group it was found to be moderate or severe in about 75 percent. Conversely when its absence had been postulated none or a slight degree was recorded in 75 percent.

Tomlinson et al. (1970) noted that arteriosclerotic dementia is overdiagnosed and Todorov et al. (1975) conclude that "the diagnosis of senile dementia has a poor specificity."

For this reason, the population characteristics of autopsy-confirmed senile dementia seems to be worthy of consideration. All these cases represent examples of clinical dementia where senile plaques and neurofibrillary tangles were found in the cerebral cortex at autopsy. Six large autopsy series appear to contain comparable information (Fuller, 1911; Uyematsu, 1923; Rothschild, 1937; Corsellis, 1962; McNenemey, 1968; Tomlinson, 1970), which is listed in Table 4. A total of 184 cases are included in these studies.

The significance of age distribution in an autopsy series has never been evaluated because there have been no complete data on the age of an autopsy population. Recently Peress et al. (1968) have reported the age distribution of 7579 autopsies in New York. Risk occurrence of senile dementia at autopsy (Table 5.5) is represented as a percentage comparison with this group. All ages represent age at the time of autopsy, which can be assumed to be roughly an average of 5 years later than age of onset. An increasing percentage of senile dementia occurs in an autopsy population until age 80–84, maintains this level through 85–89, and *declines* after 90. The sex distribution (Table 5.6) reveals an overall 2:1 female to male ratio but this sex preponderance was not present in the series of Tomlinson et al. or Fuller. The same inconsistency regarding sex is present in autopsies, as has been noted in clinical study.

Table 5.5. Age distribution of autopsy senile dementia

Author Age group	60–64	65–69	70–74	75–79	80–84	85–89	90+
Fuller (1911)	1	2	3	2	4	2	0
Uyematsu (1923)	5	6	12	14	10	8	3
Rothschild (1931)	0	6	6	5	8	2	1
Corsellis (1962)	1	6	8	14	9	7	1
McNenemey (1968)	4	2	4	5	10	7	1
Tomlinson (1970)	3	2	4	5	10	7	1
Total (autopsy)	14	24	37	42	44	27	6
Peress et al. (1968)	918	1027	822	754	574	351	112
Age risk [a]	1.5	2.3	4.5	5.6	7.7	7.7	5.4

[a] The age risk represents a percentage of the autopsy population represented by the survey of Peress et al. (1968)

Table 5.6. Sex distribution of autopsy senile dementia

Author	M	F
Corsellis (1962)	11	35
Uyematsu (1923)	15	43
Tomlinson (1970)	20	16
Rothschild (1931)	5	19
Fuller (1911)	9	5
McNenemey (1968)	–	–
Total	60	118

The GM Survey

Characteristics of the Population

This study involves a 65+ population in St. Louis, Missouri, who are domiciled in a hotel that has been remodeled as a habitus for healthy elderly persons. Varying-sized condominiums are purchased by the residents and they include food, housekeeping, and health service. The latter is not mandatory but is used at least partially by all of the residents. Nursing service is avalable 24 h daily. Two physicians comprise the medical staff, one of whom is available each morning.

The unit is located at the periphery of St. Louis, affording easy access to both St. Louis and St. Louis County. This location assumes importance because modern St. Louis has been considered to exemplify central-city population decline within the core jurisdiction of its metropolitan area (Morrison, 1974). Most of the decline is due to an exodus into St. Louis County. As a result, 20% of the white population of St. Louis is over 65 whereas the national average is 10%. Most of the residents daily enter these communities either for gainful occupation or for charitable activity.

The population is chiefly a high-middle-class white Christian society. The residents are largely single, representing surviving members of a marital unit. A majority have had some college education and about third have been self-employed professional persons or wives of such people. Almost all are former residents of St. Louis or St. Louis County but at least 65% were not born in St. Louis. Most residents have some family members living in the metropolitan area with whom they interact socially.

Methods

This investigation was conducted over a 12-month period between February 1, 1975 and January 31, 1976. It included 130 individuals who have been living at the unit during that time and 9 former residents currently in nursing homes. Ninety-nine persons were personally inverviewed for an average of 1 h during which an evaluation of dementia was completed using the dementia score of Blessed et al. (1968). The remaining 40 individuals did not consent to a personal interview but each one has been known to the medical staff for at least 1 year. A physical evaluation by one of the staff physicians was required prior to acceptance into the unit, so mental competence on admission and subsequent change were readily recognized by both physicians and nurses. None of the other 40 residents was considered to be even questionably demented.

Diagnosis of Dementia

Senile dementia was diagnosed on the basis of a history of increasing memory loss involving events (Kral, 1962), periodic or persistent confusion, disorientation as to time and place, and the occurrence of aphasia, agnosia, and apraxia. A dementia scale greater than 5 was present in each case (Blessed et al., 1968).

Acute confusion was recognized by an acute onset of persistent or recurring disorientation regarding person, time, and place. In one case this appeared to be related to hyponatremia, while in two other cases, a hip fracture was the triggering event. In each case the duration of confusion was greater than 6 months.

Creutzfeldt-Jakob disease (CJD) was diagnosed on the basis of a rapidly evolving dementia proceeding to mutism within 2 months and death after 4 months.

Normal pressure hydrocephalus (NPH) was based on a syndrome of increasing apathy, gait disturbance, urinary and fecal incontinence, and disorientation followed by improvement of all symptoms following shunt therapy.

Arteriosclerotic dementia was established on the basis of multiple strokes involving transient or permanent limb paresis or paralysis.

Results

Twenty cases of dementia have been recognized with an onset either during the year of survey or as long as 5 years prior to this interval (Table 5.7). This represents a prevalence of 14.3%, which is certainly within the range of prevalence reported in earlier surveys (Table 5.1). Early-onset dementia is screened out by the medical examination prior to acceptance into GM, so no dementia is present under the age of 74. An occurrence rate higher than that reported by Akesson, Bollerup, or Kay et al. is probably related chiefly to the age of the population. There is a much greater number of individuals aged 80+ than that occurring in the state of Missouri (Table 5.8) or in any earlier survey. There is

Table 5.7. Diagnostic characteristics of GM dementia

Normal pressure hydrocephalus (NPH)	1
Creutzfeldt-Jakob disease (CJD)	1
Arteriosclerotic dementia (AS)	2
Acute confusion (AC)	3
Senile dementia (SD)	13
Total	20

Table 5.8. Prevalence at age of onset (percentage of proband population) of all GM dementia with a comparison of GM and Missouri population over 65

Age group	Dementia		GM population over 65 (%)	Missouri population over 65 (%)
	Onset (%)	Risk [a] (%)		
65–69	0	0	0.7	34.8
70–74	0.7	9.1	7.4	27.6
75–79	3.6	19.2	17.6	16.4
80–84	5.7	14.3	33.1	12.6
85–89	3.6	17.24	18.2	5.8
90+	9.7	8.3	15.5	2.7

[a] Risk refers to a percentage of dementia among the probands of that age group only.

an increasing morbidity risk (14%–19%) between the ages of 75 and 89 but a distinct change occurred after the age of 90. Only 2 of 24 90-year-olds evinced a dementing syndrome. Therefore the contention that there is an increasing morbidity risk with increasing age does not appear to be applicable to this group of 90-year-olds. Acutally similar data can be derived from the study of Larsson et al. (1963) and from the evaluation of autopsy material (Table 5.4).

The sex distribution initially appears to support the contention of Kay et al. (1964) that senile dementia is much more common in females than in males. However the GM population is overwhelmingly female in relationship to the Missouri population. When the prevalence is corrected for sex distribution, the difference between the sexes does not appear significant either for dementia in general or for senile dementia in particular (Table 5.9.)

Table 5.9. GM senile dementia according to age and sex

	M	F	Total	Age risk (%) [a]
65–69	–	–		–
70–74	–	1	1	9.1
75–79	–	3	3	11.5
80–84	1	3	4	8.2
85–89	1	3	4	13.7
90+	–	1	1	4.2
Total	2	11		
Sex risk	7.6%	9.6%		

[a] The age risk is calculated as a percentage of the same age poupulation while the sex risk is calculated as a percentage of the same sex population.

Of course the size of this survey precludes any definite conclusion, but some interesting aspects of dementia are present.

1. Increasing age is associated with increased morbidity for dementia but only to the age of 90. This is in agreement with the study of Larsson et al. (1963).
2. Nonagenarians may represent a group that is resistant to brain disease. This concept has also been suggested by the autopsy data of Peress et al. (1968). McKeown (1975) found no plaques or tangles in 19% of 90+ brains and only 15% had arteriosclerosis.
3. Sex does not appear to be a predisposing factor in senile dementia.
4. Optimal socioeconomic status and environment do not appear to be a deterrent to the evolution of senile dementia. Incidentally, serious functional mental disorder is noted in less than 5% of the GM population and the favorable environment at GM may be an important factor in this low occurrence, since 25%–35% of 65+ population is usually considered to have such problems.
5. Further epidemiologic assays of elderly populations should involve a more complete breakdown of the 65+ population with particular attention to the 90+ group.

Etiologic Implications of Epidemiology

Aging

Most surveys have supported the aging-related concept of dementia by claiming increasing prevalence with age. When Kay reviewed epidemiologic surveys in 1972 he noted:

> All statistics and surveys agree that brain syndromes become increasingly more frequent beyond the age of 60 or 65. There seems to be a sharp rise after 90 when as many as one fifth of the population may be effected.

The paradox of this statement is that there is no attempt to break down this massive occurrence of dementia. Yet all these investigators imply that increasing morbidity continues indefinitely and, if we live long enough, everyone will be demented. Actually there is no study that demonstrates an age at which dementia is inevitable or even an increased morbidity past the age of 90. The GM survey suggests that nonagenarians may be particularly resistant to brain disease at any age. A study of this age population certainly makes more sense than a study of 70-year-olds.

Heredity

The study by Larsson et al. is the most thorough survey relating to hereditary factors in dementia. In their concluding remarks several points appear worthy of note:

> The evidence obtained concerning important hereditary factors in the etiology of senile dementia does not exclude the possibility that senile dementia is sometimes conditioned by exogenous factors, but presumably by factors that are connected with the physiological process of aging and not with "sociomedical environment".
> The enhanced morbidity risk among the relatives of senile dementia patients proves the significance of genetic factors, but the present material is not sufficient for a distinction between different possible hypotheses.
> . . . the most probable hypothesis seems to be that senile dementia is in the main conditioned by a major gene which is inherited as a monohybrid autosomal dominant.

The hereditary concept of senile dementia is immediately rendered plausible by the recognition of genetic factors in other dementing syndromes such as Huntington's chorea, hereditary forms of Alzheimer's disease (AD) and finally the early occurrence of dementia with plaques and tangles in Down's syndrome. One surprising aspect of the Larsson et al. study is that no increase in AD (dementia prior to 65) has been noted in the proband families. The results of the survey extended similar conlcusions by Constantinidis et al. (1962) and together they have prompted renewed interest in hereditary factors of AD.

The genetics of AD have been reviewed by Pratt (1970), who feels that the sporadic cases that form the bulk of the proband series are more consistent with "polygenic inheritance with a shared predisposition to Alzheimer's disease and senile dementia" rather than a single autosomal dominant gene. These cases are in distinct contrast to the much rarer examples of true familial AD in which a dominant abnormal genetic pattern has been established (Wheelan, 1959). Similar patterns have been established in Pick's disease (Malamud and Wagonner, 1943), with AD plus congophilic angiopathy (Corsellis and Brierly, 1954), dementia without plaques and tangles (Shaumberg and Suzuki, 1968), and CJD (Ferber et al., 1973).

Another curious aspect of AD genetics is that an occurrence (prior to age 65) has been noted in one but not in both monozygotic twins (Hunter et al., 1972). On the other hand Kallman (1956) has reported a concordant senile dementia rate of 43% for monozygotic twins but only 8% for dizygotic twins. To date, chromosome assays have been inconclusive. An early study by Nielsen (1968) has revealed an increase of hypo-diploid cells and later Bergener and Jungklaas (1970) have described acentric chromo-somes. However, Mark and Brun (1973) in a more recent survey could not confirm these findings and instead could find no chromosomal distinction of familial or sporadic AD from normal senescence.

Slow Virus Infection

The spread of slow virus infection has been shown to occur in various ways to form rather distinct epidemiologic patterns. In reality is was the unusual distribution of kuru that suggested an infectious etiology and prompted the initial attempt at animal trans-mission. The mode of spread in kuru was by the oral route, since the cannibalism of the Fore tribesmen involved ingestion of the brain of deceased members of the tribe. Oral transmission as well as contact spread of scrapie to sheep and goats has also been reported (Pattison and Millson, 1961; Brotherson et al., 1968).

Several epidemiologic surveys of CJD have appeared recently (Bobowick et al., 1973; Matthews, 1975; Kahana et al., 1973). While no distinct modes of transmission have been demonstrated, several important findings have been noted in these studies and in other case reports.

1. There is an extraordinary occurrence of CJD in Libyan Jews with an incidence of 31.3 per million as opposed to 0.4—1.9 per million for other ethnic groups in Israel.
2. Bobowick et al suggested that ingestion of hog brain might have etiologic significance, since one-third of his cases gave a history of such dietary habit. However, a similar number of his controls had a similar history, albeit without the same frequency. Matthewsdid not find support for this concept in his study.
3. Some geographic clustering was reported by Matthews and Mayer et al. (1977) but not by Bobowick et al.
4. Most cases appear to be sporadic although a new familial case was discovered by Bobowick et al.
5. At least two definite examples of human transmisssion of CJD have been reported. The first involved a corneal transplant from a person who died from disease (Duffy et al., 1974). The second episode involved the reuse of an electrode that had been implanted on a patient with DJD (Manuelides et al., 1977). In this case sterilization in 70% alcohol and formaldehyde vapor was not effective and spongiform encephalo-pathy occurred in two subsequent cases.
6. Animal transmission in two cases of hereditary forms of CJD suggests that the trans-missible agent has some chromosomal linkage but this has not been clarified by cur-rent study (Ferber et al., 1973). It is interesting to note that the two cases of trans-missible AD were also examples of hereditary disease.

Concluding Remarks

The potential of epidemiology as a determinant of dementia is confirmed dramatically by the studies of kuru but it has not been realized in senile dementia. Nonetheless some intriguing aspects of the problem have been revealed or intimated by these studies. Some familial influence on sporadic occurrence is indicated by Larsson et al. (1963) and Constantinidis et al. (1962) but this appears to be distinct from the autosomal dominance that is present in true familial cases. The marked difference in prevalence in different populations that is revealed by the epidemiologic studies, such as those of Akesson and Nielsen, could be the result of differing individual or environmental predisposition, but a more uniform system of assay is needed to establish these concepts. An intriguing resistance to dementia after the age of 90 is suggested by the GM survey, the Larsson et al. study, and by the autopsy cases, but a study specifically relating to this age group is needed to clarify this idea.

References

Austin, D.F., Werner, S.B. (1974): Epidemiology for the Health Sciences. Springfield: C.C. Thomas

Akesson, H.O. (1969): A population study of senile and arterisclerotic psychoses. Hum. Hered. 19, 546–566

Bell, L.U. (1844): Twenty-sixth annual report of the McLean Asylum for the Insane. Boston: James Loring Press

Bergener, M., Jungklaas, F.K. (1970): Genetische Befunde bei Morbus Alzheimer und seniler Demenz. Gerontal. Clin. 12, 71–75

Bevan Lewis, W. (1899): A Textbook of Mental Diseases. London: Charles Griffin

Blandford, G.F. (1878): Insanity and its Treatment. Edinburgh: Oliver and Boyd

Blessed, G., Tomlinson, B.E., Roth, M. (1968): The association between quantitative measures of dementia and of senile change in the cerebral gray matter of elderly subjects. Br. J. Psychiatry 114, 797–811

Bobowick, A.R., Brody, J.A., Matthews, M.R., Roos, R., Gajdusek, D.C. (1973): Creutzfeldt-Jakob disease: A case control study. Am. J. Epidemiol. 98, 381–394

Bollerup, T.R. (1975): Prevalence of mental illness among 70 year olds domiciled in nine Copenhagen suburbs. Acta Psychiatr. Scand. 51, 327–340

Brotherson, J.G., Renwick, C.C., Stamp, J.T., Zlotnik, I. (1968): Spread of scrapie by contact to goats and sheep. J. Comp. Pathol. 78, 9–17

Constantinidis, J., Garrone, G., Ajuriaguerra, J. (1962): L'hérédité des démences de l'age avancé. L'Encephale 51, 301–344

Corsellis, J.A.N., Brierly, J.B. (1954): An unusual type of presenile dementia. Brain 77, 571–585

Corsellis, J.A.N. (1962): Mental Illness and the Aging Brain. London: Oxford University

Duffy, P., Wolf, J., Collins, G., DeVoe, A.G., Streeten, B., Cowen, D. (1974): Possible person-to-person transmission of Creutzfeldt-Jakob disease. N. Engl. J. Med. 290, 692–693

Essen-Moller, E. (1956): Individual traits and morbidity in a Swedish rural population. Acta Psychiatr. Scand. (Suppl.) 100

Ferber, R.A., Wiesenfeld, S.L., Roos, R.P., Bobowick, Gibbs, C.J., Jr., Gajdusek, D.C. (1973): Familial Creutzfeldt-Jakob disease: Transmission of the familial disease to primates. Proc. X Int. Cong. Neurol. Int. Cong. Series No. 319. Amsterdam: Excerpta Medica, pp. 358–380

Fuller, S. (1911): A study of miliary plaques found in brains of the aged. Am. J. Ins. 68, 10–217

Gruenberg, E.M. (1959): A mental health survey of older persons. In: Comparative Epidemiology of the Mental Disorders. Hoch, P.H., Zubin, J. (eds.). New York: Grune and Stratton, pp. 13–23

Hagnell, O. (1970): Disease expectancy and incidence of mental illness among the aged. Acta Psychiatr. Scand. 46 (Suppl. 219), 83–89

Hunter, R., Dayan, A.D., Wilson, J. (1972): Alzheimer's disease in one monozygotic twin. J. Neurol. Neurosurg. Psychiatry 35, 707–710

Kahana, E., Alter, M., Braham, J., Sofer, D. (1974): Creutzfeldt-Jakob disease: Focus among Lybian Jews in Israel. Science 183, 90–91

Kallman, F.J. (1956): Genetic aspects of mental disorders in later life. In: Mental Disorders in Later Life. Kaplan, O.J. (ed.). Stanford: Standord Univ., pp. 26–46

Kay, D.W.K., Beamish, P., Roth, M. (1964): Old age mental disorders in Newcastle upon Tyne. Br. J. Psychiatry 110, 146–148

Kay, D.W.K. (1972): Epidemiological aspects of organic brain disease in the aged. In: Aging and the Brain. Gaitz, C.M. (ed.). New York: Plenum, pp. 15–27

Kral, V.A. (1962): Senescent forgetfulness, benign and malignant. Can. Med. Assoc. J. 86, 257–260

Larsson, T., Sjogren, T., Jacobson, G. (1963): Senile dementia. Acta Psychiatr. Scand. 39 (Suppl. 167), 1–227

Malamud, N., Wagonner, R.W. (1943): Genealogic and clinico pathologic study of Pick's disease. Arch. Neurol. Psychiatry 50, 288–303

Manuelides, E.E., Angelo, J.N., Gorgacz, E.J., Manuelides, L. (1977): Danger of accidental person-to-person transmission of Creutzfeldt-Jakob disease by surgery. Lancet 1, 478–479

Mark, J., Brun, A. (1973): Chromosomal deviations in Alzheimer's disease compared to those in senescence and senile dementia. Gerontol. Clin. 15, 253–258

Matthews, W.B. (1975): Epidemiology of Creutzfeldt-Jakob disease in England and Wales. J. Neurol. Neurosurg. Psychiatry 38, 210–213

Mayer, V., Orolin, D., Mitrova, E. (1977): Cluster of Creutzfeldt-Jakob disease and presenile dementia. Lancet 2, 256

McKeown, E.F. (1975): De Senectute: The F.E. Williams Lecture. J. R. Coll. Physicians Lond. 10, 79–99

McMenemey, W.H. (1968): Present concepts of Alzheimer's disease. In: Central Nervous System. Some Experimental Models of Neurological Disease. Bailey, O.T., Smith, D.E. (eds.). Baltimore: Williams and Wilkins, pp. 201–208

Morrison, P.A. (1974): Urban growth and decline: San Jose and St. Louis in the 1960's. Science 185, 757–762

Nielsen, J. (1962): Geronto-psychiatric period-prevalence investigation in a geographically delimited population. Acta Psychiatr. Scand. 38, 307–330

Nielsen, J. (1968): Chromosomes in senile dementia. Br. J. Psychiatry 114, 303–309

Pattison, I.H., Millson, G.C. (1961): Experimental transmission of scrapie to goats and sheep by the oral route. J. Comp. Pathol. Therap. 71, 171–176

Peress, N.S., Kone, W.C., Aronson, S.M. (1968): Central nervous system findings in a tenth decade autopsy population. In: Alzheimer's Disease and Related Disorders. Wolstenholme, G.E.W., O'Connor, M. (eds.). London: Churchill, pp. 473–483

Pratt, R.T.C. (1970): The genetics of Alzheimer's disease. In: Alzheimer's Disease and Related Disorders. Wolstenholme, G.E.W., O'Connor, M. (eds.). London: Churchill, pp. 137–139

Roth, M. (1955): The natural history of mental disorder in old age. J. Ment. Sci. 101, 281–301

Rothschild, D. (1937): Pathologic changes in senile psychoses and their psychobiologic significance. Am.J. Psychiatry 93, 757–785

Shaumberg, H.H., Suzuki, K. (1968): Non-specific familial presenile dementia. J. Neurol. Neurosurg. Psychiatry 31, 479–486

Todorov, A.B., Go, R.C.P., Constantinidis, J., Elston, R.C. (1975): Specificity of the clinical diagnosis of dementia. J. Neurol. Sci. 26, 81–98

Tomlinson, B.E., Blessed, G., Roth, M. (1970): Observations on the brains of demented old people. J. Neurol. Sci. 11, 205–242

Uyematsu, S. (1923): On the pathology of senile psychosis. The differential diagnostic significance of Redlich-Fischer's miliary plaques. J. Nerv. Ment. Dis. 57, 1-25, 131–156, 243–260

Vernon, P.E. (1947): The variations of intelligence with occupation, age and locality. Br. J. Psychol. Stat. Sect. 1, 52–63

Warthin, A.S. (1928): The pathology of the aging process. Bull. N.Y.Acad. Med. 4, 1006–1046

Wheelan, L. (1959): Familial Alzheimer's disease. Ann. Human Genet. 23, 300–310

6. Current Evaluation of Pathologic Correlates of Dementia

The involvement of pathology in mental disease was confirmed by Wilks in 1864:

> The more marked changes which have been described as occurring in the insane, especially in those long demented, are those of an atrophic kind; the whole brain, when weighed, is found to be much lighter than an organ would be which had quite filled the skull case.
>
> Thus on removing the dura mater, the surface of the brain is often quite hidden by the layer of serum which lies beneath the arachnoid, and filling up the spaces between the convolutions; instead of the sulci meeting they are widely separated, and their intervals filled with serum, and which, on being removed with the pia mater, the full depth of the sulci can be seen, At the same time the ventricles are distended by a large amount of serum; their walls are granular and the choroid plexus is full of cysts.
>
> Such conditions are indicative of a wasted brain and are those which have been regarded as characteristic of a chronic form of insanity.

This is the change in the brain organ which is the basis for all concepts of "organic dementia". A consistent pathologic doctrine has been maintained since that time; the etiologic cause of the atrophy is the cause of the dementia. Unfortunately, this creed was questioned when the cellular pathology of Virchow, the improved histology of Bielschowsky, and the new histochemistry of Divry did not reveal the origin of dementia. Jervis and Soltz (1936) dismissed pathology as a determinant of dementia but they should have repudiated the technology not the concept, which is as valid today as it was for Wilks.

We have noted in Chapter 1 how the microscopic correlates of atrophy are not specific for dementia. This is an extremely important point to remember. During the last 20 years a whole new concept of cell biology has evolved as a result of the new technology; electron microscopy, biochemistry, histochemistry, and nuclear medicine. These tools have been used to reevaluate the nature of senile plaques (SP), neurofibrillary tangles (NF), granulovacuolar degeneration, and vascular disease. This has been accomplished and there is a greater appreciation of their biologic significance but their relationship to dementia has not changed. SP have the same specificity for dementia that they had 70 years ago. The new biology will be important only if new concepts of cause can be derived.

Congophilic Angiopathy

Congophilic angiopathy (CA) is an unusual, clinically unappreciated vascular disease in which amyloid is deposited in arterioles, capillaries, and venules. The term amyloid was devised by Virchow (1860) to describe certain abnormal tissue aggregates that had staining properties similar to starch. Virchow realized that this was a complex material:

"Owing to this multiplicity of reactions it is really still very difficult to say with certainty to what class the substance belongs." Nevertheless two distinct forms were recognized: primary amyloidosis due to some unknown endogenous factor, and secondary amyloidosis, which was linked to certain chronic diseases such as tuberculosis or osteomyelitis. Amyloid had an affinity for Congo red dye and, in the brain, the term congophilic angiopathy derives from this property.

The first description of probable CA was by Fischer (1910) who described thickened arterioles with a radial extension into the brain of a substance that stained metachromatically with toluidine blue. There was no systematic study of this material until Divry (1927) indentified it as amyloid on the basis of green birefringence in polarized light following Congo red staining. This discovery did not cause great interest because of the diverse nature of brain amyloid. Generalized amyloidosis had always excited pathologists but the brain did not partake in generalized amyloidosis. It was even more mysterious to have brain involvement without other organ involvement (McKeown, 1965). This cynicism was augmented by the peculiar enthusiasm of Divry and somewhat later of Schwartz. After 25 years of study Divry (1952) talks about amyloid in the following words, which border on mysticism:

Amyloid degeneration thus occurs in the senile or presenile brain (Alzheimer's disease) on the level of the senile plates *sensu stricto* of Alzheimer's degeneration and of degeneration of the vascular system.

Let us mention as a general theory, that amyloid of senile plates as well as of the vessels has sharp antixenic reactions, mainly microglia and macroglia: we must stress on the other hand that the trichosic substance is neutral in this respect; it does not appear to markedly alter the architectonic nor the structure of the figured elements in the tissue it involves.

It is proved that amyloid degeneration is an infiltration process of the invaded tissue; it is a precipitation issued from the colloidal interstitial medium; the transformation of a sol into a gel.

Divry regarded vascular deposits, SP, and NF as interrelated aspects of cerebral amyloidosis. Very few pathologists (neuro- or otherwise) were willing to accept this concept. One who did was Schwartz, who used a fluorescent dye, thioflavin, to identify amyloid. The specificity of this dye for amyloid had been questioned repeatedly, so caution seemed to be indicated in the interpretation of the widespread fluorescence that he demonstrated in aging and dementia (Schwartz, 1970). Instead, one reads some of the most flamboyant rhetoric in medical literature:

Our investigations have disclosed amyloidosis to be one of the most frequent diseases of the human species, and cerebral amyloidosis, because of its enormous incidence in the aged, to be the most important condition in neuropathology!

Amyloidosis is of paramount importance in the causation of psychiatric and neurologic conditions.

Amyloidosis, as things presently stand, seems to be an inevitable condition. Living long enough, no human being escapes it.

By 1970 very few neuropathologists outside Germany believed that CA had any etiologic significance for plaques, for dementia, or for any other brain dysfunction. True amyloidosis is uncommon, so most pathologists had very little experience with this condition; furthermore they did not believe Divry and Schwartz. The unfortunate aspect of all this confusion is that some careful and more modest investigators were also reporting on the problem but they were being submerged. The most important of these men was Sholz (1938), who demonstrated two forms of vascular amyloid. Amyloid could be seen to be confined within the walls of small arteries, especially in the meninges and the superficial cortex. This pattern seems to be more common and it can exist independently in mild degrees of involvement. In arterioles and capillaries, the amyloid was not limited to the vascular wall but also showed numerous projections into the adjacent brain (Fig. 6.1), which were invariably associated with perivascular SP. The small-vessel involvement has been called "drüsige Entartung der Arterien and Capillaren" by Sholz (1938) and "dyshoric angiopathy" by Morel and Wildi (1952). Only this microangiopathic form appears to have relevance for dementia.

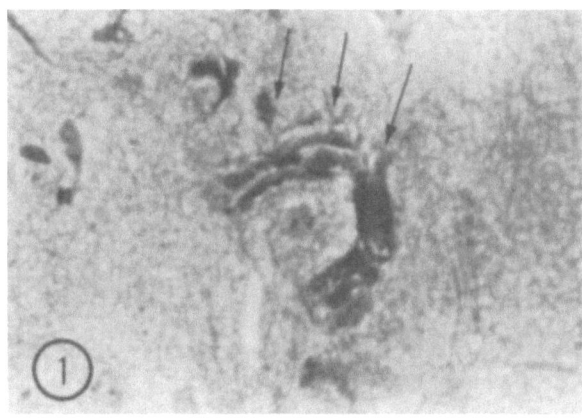

Fig. 6.1. Light micrograph of a blood vessel in the cerebral cortex in which abnormal material (PAS positive) occurs in the vascular wall and extends into the adjacent brain (*arrows*). LFB/PAS x 800

The occurrence of CA microangiopathy seems to be greater in Europe if the medical reports can be considered an indicator of its incidence. Two distinct forms have been recognized: familial and sporadic. The familial disease had been observed initially by Worster-Drought et al. (1940) and since that time six other cases have been reported (Table 6.1). Early onset with slow progression and no sex prevalence is noted in these people. A clinical syndrome of progressive dementia is accompanied by some combination of dysarthria, spastic limb paralysis, and ataxic gait. Involvement of the cerebral cortex can be associated with similar findings in Ammon's horn, cerebellum and basal ganglia especially the striatum. The SP are chiefly perivascular and, although NF are present in each case, they are not as widely distributed as the plaques.

Sporadic disease has been reported by several investigators (Table 6.2) and the great disparity of information renders comparison impossible except for age at death. These sporadic cases seem to have a much later occurrence than the familial involvement. Clinically all except two appear to have been demented (Neumann, 1960; Torack, 1975). The largest series by far is that of Morel and Wildi (1952) who have made the following pathologic observations: (1) The degree of atrophy is similar to senile dementia but much less than that of AD (dementia under 65). (2) The occipital lobes are involved predominantly and on occasion, exclusively. (Author's note: The cortical involvement can be very selective involving only layers II and IV, as noted originally by Lowenberg in 1928). (3) Perivascular senile plaques are present in every case but neurofibrillary tangles are present in only 25% of all cases. (4) No amyloid is present in tissues other than brain. Two other findings appear to be worthy of mention. Ulrich (1972) and

Table 6.1. Familial occurrence of congophilic angiopathy

Reference	Sex	Age Onset	Death	Clinical symptoms	Family dementia	Vascular distribution	Senile plaques	Neurofibrillary tangles
Worster-Drought et al. (1940)	Male	47	54	Dysarthria, progressive dementia, spastic paralysis, ataxic gait	11 in 3 generations	Pial, cortical white matter	Ammon's horn, cerebellum, cerebral white matter	Ammons's horn
Worster-Drought et al. (1944)	Female	44	51	Progressive dementia, dysarthria, ataxia, spastic paresis (arms)	Sibling of No. 1	Pial, cortical white matter	Ammons's horn, cerebellum, brain stem	Ammon's horn
Corsellis and Brierly (1954) Case 1	Female	51	54	Progressive dementia, spastic paresis	Mother D. 55 brother D. 40	Cortical and pial	Cerebral cortex, Ammon's horn, striatum	Cerebral cortex, Ammon's horn
Corsellis and Brierly (1954) Case 2	Female	56	66	Progressive dementia, spasticity of all limbs	Mother D.?	Cortical and pial	Cerebral cortex	Cerebral cortex
Van Bogaert et al. (1940)	Male	25	39	Spastic paraplegia, progressive dementia, dysarthria, ataxic gait	2 siblings (similar age)	Cortical	Cerebral cortex, striatum cerebellum	Cerebral cortex, Ammon's horn
Luers (1947)	Male	26	41	Spastic paraplegia, progressive dementia, dysarthria	Sister	Cortical and pial	Cerebral cortex, Ammon's horn, striatum cerebellum	Cerebral cortex,
Gerhard et al. (1972)	Female	45	47	Dysarthria, progressive dementia	Mother, grandfather	Cerebral cortex, meninges	Cerebral cortex, striatum, thalamus	Cerebral cortex, striatum

Table 6.2. Reports of sporadic congophilic angiopathy

Author	Number of cases	Age at death
Morel and Wildi (1952)	34	58–91
Neumann (1960)	1	45
Hollander and Strich (1968)	6	55–69
Ulrich et al. (1973)	5	52–74
Mandybur et al. (1975)	4	61–83
Torack (1975)	3	62–76
Jellinger (1977)	15	64–86

Gerhard (1973) mention a prominent history of rheumatoid arthritis in the patients and in their families. Cerebral hemorrhage seems to be quite common and Seitelberger (1974), Torack (1975), and Jellinger (1977) have stressed CA as a cause of hemorrhage in the elderly.

The impact of all these studies was minimized because no one knew what amyloid was or why it was made. Pathologists have believed, in agreement with Virchow, that vascular amyloid is derived from the circulation. The perivascular spikes of amyloid surrounding brain capillaries have been interpreted to indicate leaky blood vessels that allow an amyloid factor to affect the vessel wall and to enter the brain. The demonstration by Glenner et al. (1971) that amyloid is composed of immunoglobulins derived from the circulation reinforced these ideas and gave new meaning to the amyloid topic.

Electron-microscopic study of biopsy material has confirmed the presence of amyloid in these blood vessels (Schlote, 1965; Torack, 1975). In each case extracellular fibrils, 90 Å in thickness, have been demonstrated within vascular walls. Arteriolar, capillary, and venular involvement has been studied by Torack (1975) and the changes in endothelial (Fig. 6.2) and perithelial cells (Fig. 6.3) have been considered compatible with an exogenous (circulating) source of amyloid precursor. Perivascular plaque amyloid is contiguous with vascular amyloid (Figs. 6.4–6.7). Relatively few thickened neurites were present around these cores of amyloid. A most intriguing aspect of this study is the sequential comparison of cortex in biopsy with the autopsy 8 days later in one case. There was a dramatic increase in thickened neurites and characteristic "mature" SP in the autopsy (Figs. 6.8, 6.9).

There are many aspects of amyloid microangiopathy that would argue for distinction from AD: (1) A familial form with early onset, slow progression, a clinical syndrome distinguished by dementia with dysarthria, spastic paralysis, and ataxia and finally by pathologic changes in the cerebellum. (2) Specificity of the vascular response is indicated in sporadic disease by the occipital lobe involvement and by the rare laminar distribution but most impressive is the array of amyloid around small vascular structures, which occurs in no other disorder. (3) A rather unique tissue response in which there is a constant relationship to perivascular SP but in sporadic cases only an infrequent (25%) relationship to NF. It seems appropriate to consider amyloid microangiopathy as an etiologically unique form of human dementia.

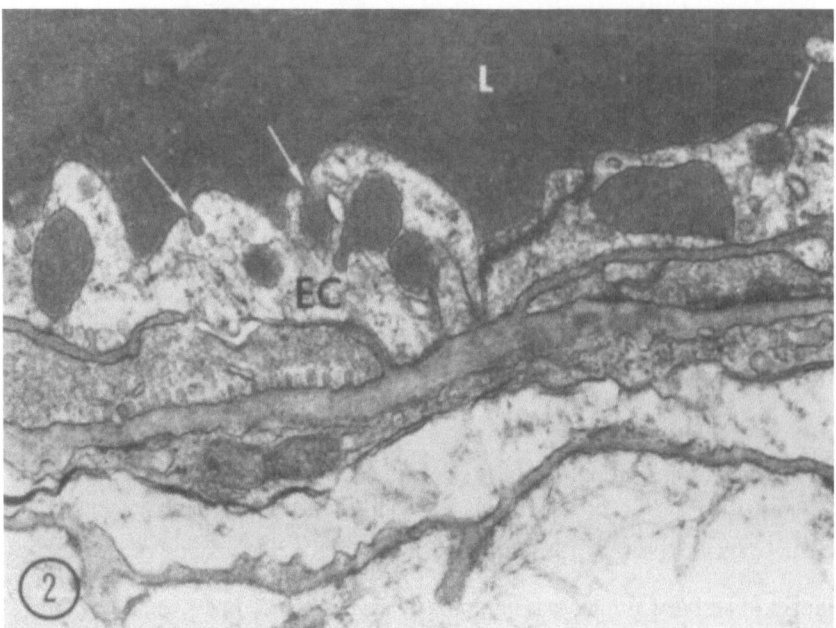

Fig. 6.2. Electron micrograph of a probable venule in which the endothelial cell (*EC*) has numerous varying sized vesicles containing material having the same electron density as the plasma in the lumen. Some of these vesicles communicate with the lumen (*L*) (*arrows*). x 9000

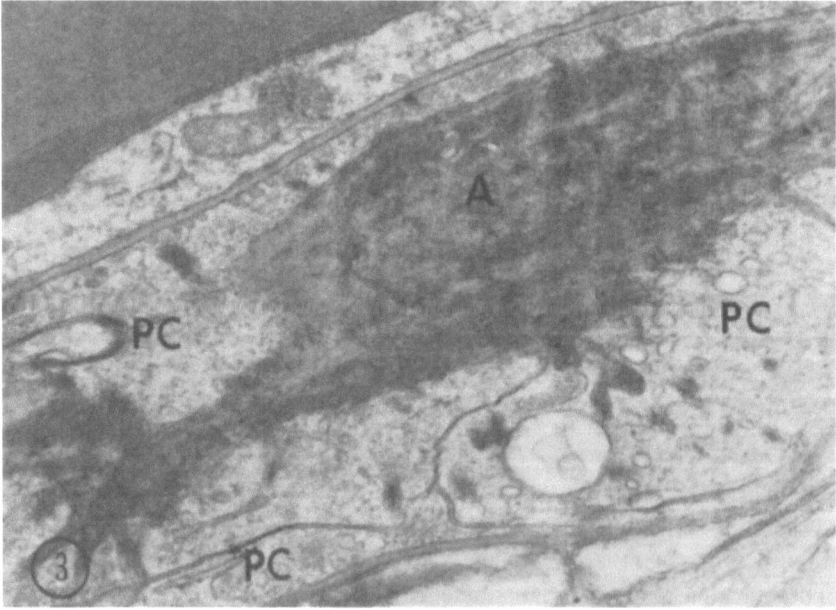

Fig. 6.3. Electron micrograph of the wall of a blood vessel (? venule) in which three perithelial cells (*PC*) can be identified. In the extracellular space between two of these an irregular mass of fibrillar material is seen, the fibers of which are compatible with amyloid (*A*). There are numerous extensions of such material into the cytoplasm of these cells, which is similar to that of Kupffer cells producing amyloid. x 8000

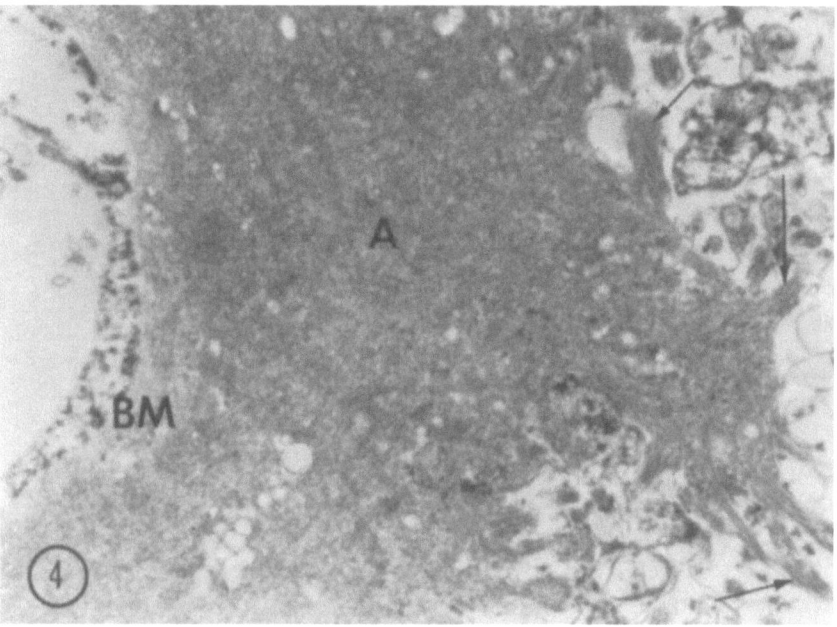

Fig. 6.4. Electron micrograph of a blood vessel in which the amyloid (A) is continuous with the basement membrane area (BM) and extends into the adjacent brain extracellular spaces. The projections (arrows) are very reminiscent of the pattern of deposition between pericytes seen in Figure 3. x 5000

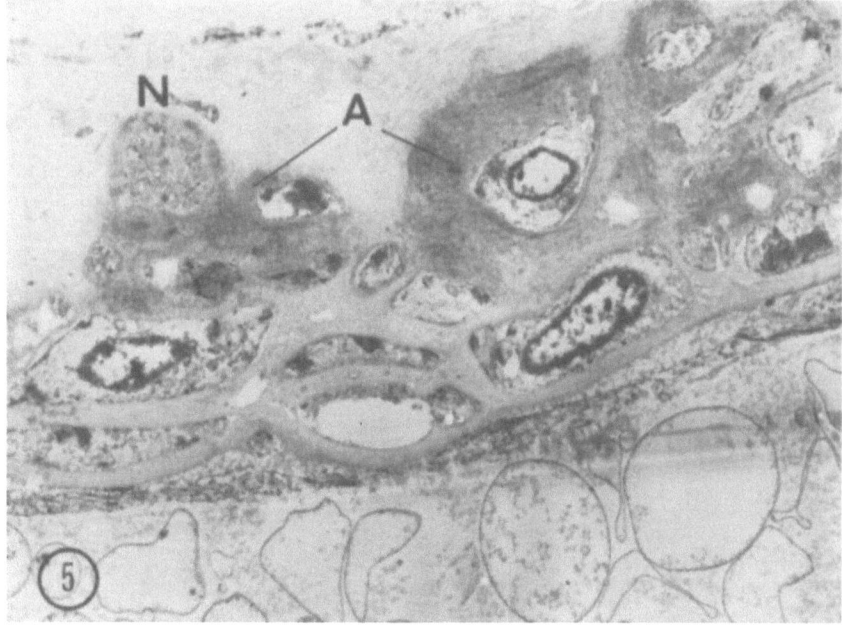

Fig. 6.5. Electron micrograph of a vascular wall in which amyloid deposition (A) has a distinct pericellular organization. At least one of these can be identified as a neurite (N). x 2500

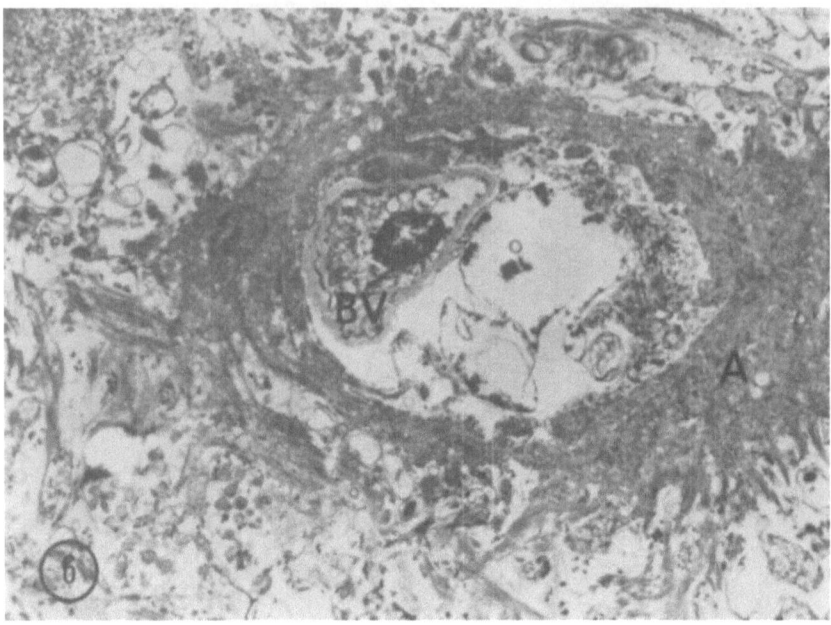

Fig. 6.6. Electron micrograph of a blood vessel (*BV*), which is completely surrounded by a mass of amyloid (*A*). x 2000

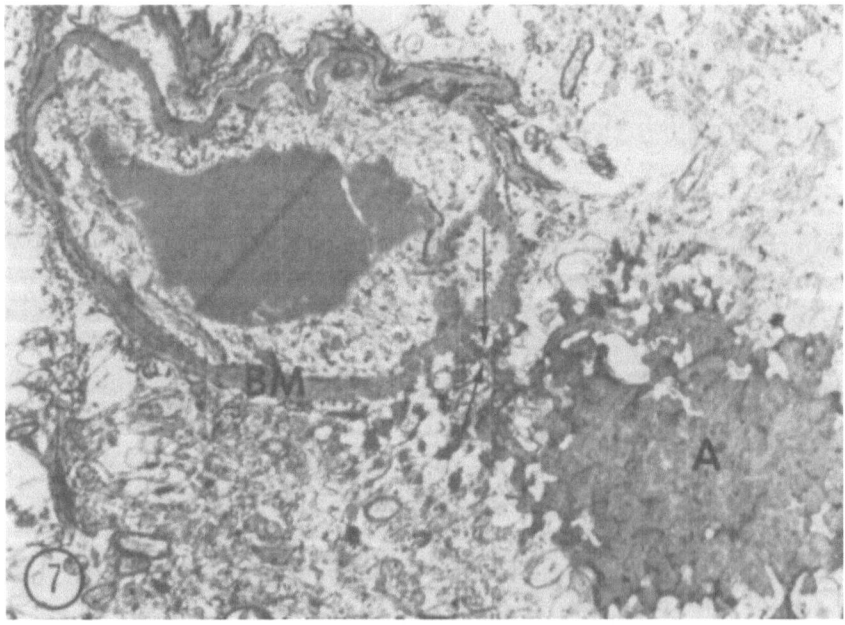

Fig. 6.7. A perivascular plaque, which has only a single point of continuity between the amyloid mass (*A*) and the basement membrane (*BM*) (*arrows*). x 3000

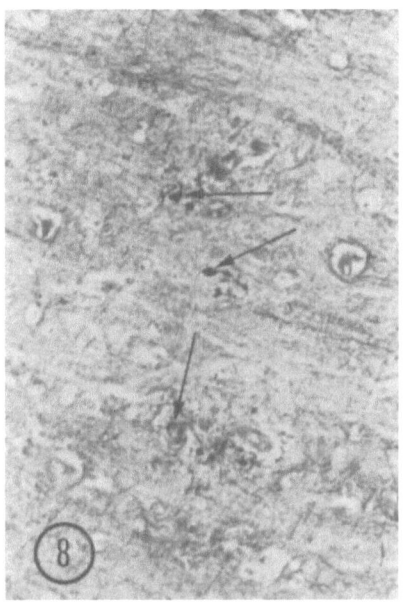 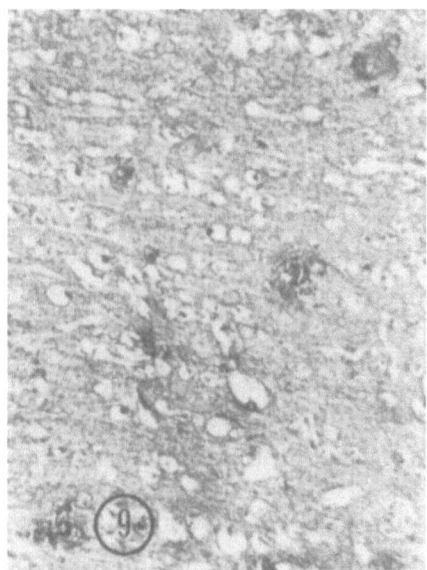

Fig. 6.8   Fig. 6.9

Fig. 6.8. Light micrograph of brain biopsy in a patient with CA. There are several foci of thickened neurites (*arrows*) but not distinct plaque formation is visible. Sevier x 300

Fig. 6.9. Light micrograph of brain parenchym adjacent to the biopsy site 8 days after the biopsy procedure. Numerous well-developed senile plaques in contrast to the appearance in Figure 6.8. Sevier x 200

Senile Plaques

In 1911 Fuller wrote a detailed and astute report from his own experience and the knowledge then current about the nature of SP, which except for some minor additions constituted what we knew about plaques for the next 50 years. (1) The distribution is chiefly in the cerebral cortex, especially the frontal and temporal lobes, but they occur on occasion in basal ganglia, white matter, brain stem, and cerebellum. (2) The core of the plaque consisted of an amorphous extracellular material, which was considered to be the result of a primary glial reaction to the injurious agent. (3) The periphery of the plaque was composed of thickened neurites with an admixture of fibrous astrocytes. (4) A relationship to blood vessels was noted but this was not consistent enough to suggest a vascular origin. Only the identification of microglia by Ley in 1922 and of amyloid in 1927 by Divry were meaningful additions to Fuller's knowledge.

The surprising aspect of SP is that a major role in the evolution of dementia has not been stressed until recently. We have noted how Alzheimer was not impressed with plaques because he thought they were glial in origin. Their frequent occurrence in non-demented elderly was another reason for not ascribing importance to them. Finally there was no agreement as to the origin of these unusual structures. The first 38 years of plaque investigation were reviewed very ably by Ferraro (1931), who summarizes this exercise with these words:

As may be seen from this rapid survey of the literature concerning the histogenesis of the senile plaque, no agreement seems to exist as to the origin of such a lesion; one group of investigators favors the theory that it originates from nerve cells, another, that it originates from the neuroglial elements, another, from axis cylinders, and still another, from the intercellular ground substance.

A new appreciation of the importance of SP was stimulated by the studies of Tomlinson et al. (1970). SP were more prominent than NF in mild cases of dementia and they were much more common in the nondemented elderly (Tomlinson et al., 1968). Equally impressive is the occurrence of SP as early as the third decade whereas NF do not appear until the fourth decade (Tomlinson, 1977). Perhaps the most significant observation was that an SP count of 14 or more per low-power field was a consistent indicator of definite dementia. Once again the NF were more variable. These findings have been confirmed at least in the hippocampus by Morimatsu et al. (1975). The pathologic implications of these findings are threefold: (1) A distinct morphologic criterion of dementia has been demonstrated. (2) The SP rather than the NF is the primary abnormality of this dementing process. (3) There is no qualitative distinction between aging and dementia.

When Terry et al. (1964), Krigman et al. (1965), and Kidd (1964) described the ultrastructure of SP, the new cell biology was applied to understand plaque formation. The amyloid core was confirmed by the occurrence of 90-Å extracellular filaments indentical to those that had been described previously in systemic amyloidosis (Cohen and Calkins, 1959). The thickened neurites represented dendrites and small axons dilated by masses of filaments, dense bodies, or mitochondria. This was the kind of axon reaction that Weiss (1961) was talking about when he obstructed axon flow. The glial component was of two types. One glial cell had a relationship to the amyloid and this was considered to be a microglial cell that was producing the amyloid. The second glial cell, a fibrous astrocyte, was believed to be a reactive cell. All that remained to complete the ultrastructure was the description of altered synapses by Gonatas et al. in 1967.

Histochemical studies after Divry related chiefly to enzyme histochemistry. Elevated oxidative activity (Friede, 1965; Johnson and Blum, 1970; Krigman et al., 1965) probably relates to mitochondrial packing of neurites and the increased acid phosphatase (Sizuki and Terry, 1967; Josephy, 1949) should correspond to the numerous dense bodies seen in neurites and also in nearby cell bodies. The biochemistry of plaques was indefinite until the isolation of plaques by Nikaido et al. (1971). Previously Suzuki et al. (1965) had related the increased acid polysaccharide in biopsy assay to amyloid deposition. Now the cores were separated by sonication and the chemistry of the amyloid was clarified. Unfortunately the critical information was not forthcoming from these studies. This involves a purification of the amyloid with a sequential assay of amino acid composition to determine if it is of immunoglobulin origin (Glenner et al., 1971). These studies have revealed an increased silicone content of plaques (Austin et al., 1973), but no aluminum has been noted.

Following the acquisition of this new information, it seemed logical to reevaluate the dynamics of plaque formation. Since the pathogenesis of plaques had never been established, this really involved a reappraisal of the older theories of histogenesis.

1. The neuronal origin of plaques. The frequency of cortical location, the inclusion of neurites into the periphery of the plaque, and the association with NF in neurons were arguments in favor of a primary change in neurons. According to this concept the neuron was the cellular target of an injury that caused the neurofibrillary reaction. When the cell died the cell debris (including the NF) formed the nidus of the SP.

Despite the attractiveness of this theory, few people felt that nerve cells alone were responsible for plaques.

2. The glial origin of plaques. Both Redlich (1898) and Alzheimer (1940) favored an origin of plaques based upon glial disease. Their silver impregnation primarily stained glial cells so they were always recognized to be prominent components of plaques. Oligodendrocytes and microglia were both identified as initially injured cells. The identification of some of these as oligodendroglia was due probably to the difficulty of the Hortega impregnation in separating them from microglia. The loss of these nurse cells was considered to change neuronal activity and the glial matrix following degeneration was the stimulus for the plaque development.

3. Amyloid theory. The identification of amyloid by Divry (1927) revived the concept that the plaque was due to a local deposition of a metabolic substance that was also either toxic to nerve cells or produced injury by compression atrophy.

4. Vascular theory. The inconsistent relationship between plaques and blood vessels caused this to be the least popular concept. Only in Europe, where congophilic angiopathy seems to be more common, was a vascular origin of plaques seriously considered. Dyshoric angiopathy (drüsige Entartung) was the vascular lesion that allowed this toxic material (amyloid) to enter the brain to form plaques.

None of the new studies have shown that oligodendroglia or neuronal cell bodies participate in plaque formation. The astrocytes are believed to be present as a reactive cell. The thickened neurites are due to a disruption of axon flow with an accumulation of organelles, which ordinarily move down these neurites. The altered synapses could be due to altered axon flow or to a direct involvement by the agent that effected this change. The microglia are considered to be the source of the amyloid but some substrate protein is required for its production (Glenner et al., 1973). This could be either circulating immunoglobulin or endogenous fibrous protein found in the brain. This means that plaques can represent purely a local response of that they are due to an exogenous factor in the circulation.

Endogenous Plaque Formation

The neurofibrillary mass in neuronal cell bodies constitutes the most obvious local source of a fibrous protein, yet neuron death is not considered to be the likely initial event in plaque evolution. Theoretically there is no reason why this could not happen. The dying cell could liberate its load of fibrous protein, which would be engulfed subsequently by microglia and then chopped up into the smaller pieces we call amyloid. Probably the chief argument against this concept is the lack of plaques in diseases like the amyotrophic lateral sclerosis-dementia-Parkinson complex of Guam (Hirano et al., 1961) and boxer brains (Corsellis et al., 1973), in which numerous NF are present.

The terminal end of the neuron, namely dendrites, terminal axons, and synapses are considered to be the primary site of neuronal involvement in plaques, hence the proposal to call this a neuritic plaque (Wisniewski and Terry, 1973). The major argument for this theory is that a plaque that has thickened neurites but no amyloid is the earliest plaque form. In this concept, amyloid is formed later to form a mature plaque (neuritic and amyloid content) and the cycle ends when the neurites have degenerated leaving behind the amyloid pile. The source of substrate would be the filamentous material that aggregates in the neurites probably secondary to some block of axon of dendritic flow. The theory is attractive and lacks only an explanation of how an agent inhibiting cytoplasmic transport can have such a localized effect.

Exogenous Origin From Circulating Immunoproteins

Both immunoglobulins and a serum albumen (SA) are recognized sources of amyloid substrate in human and experimental disease (Glenner et al., 1973). The presence of amyloid within the walls of the microcirculation in congophilic angiopathy duplicates the vascular changes found in other tissues. The presence of perivascular plaques with little or no neuritic involvement suggests that amyloid deposition is related to the vascular change and is a primary event (Torack, 1975). A major difficulty is the singular lack of brain amyloidosis in generalized amyloidosis, either human or experimental. This brain sparing has been explained as a function of the blood-brain barrier, which excludes macromolecules, like immunoglobulins, from entry into the brain. Therefore some disruption of this limited permeability would be necessary, perhaps analogous to that which has been shown to occur in experimental allergic encephalitis.

The proof of these theories is probably impossible in man, since the sequential events of plaque formation require an experimental model rather than the single-point study afforded by human autopsy. Alternatively SP have been studied in both aged dogs and monkeys (Wisniewski et al., 1970; Wisniewski et al., 1973a). In both species the plaques were chiefly perivascular with extensive vascular amyloid, and a subdued neuritic change. When thickened neurites were present they were dendritic and axonal with no abnormal neurofibrils. These plaques seem to be typical of those found in congophilic angiopathy.

Experimental induction of plaques has been reported in rabbits treated with aluminum especially when this was combined with an undercutting of the cortex to induce greater neuritic injury (Wisniewski and Terry, 1968). In these animals neuritic plaques without amyloid were found and this was considered argument in favor of the neuritic origin of plaque formation. Neuritic plaques with amyloid were reported most recently in mice infected with scrapie (Wisniewski et al., 1975). This is the first experimental model of amyloid deposition in the brain that has been noted at vascular walls and in perivascular plaques. In these animals, a most interesting observation is the active deposition of amyloid at the site of a stab wound. This seems to offer evidence of a circulating precursor for brain amyloid, and these early studies suggest that amyloid formation and neuritic changes occur concomitantly (Wisniewski, 1975). If these experimental models are proven correct, they would demonstrate that SP can originate either from an endogenous mechanism (neuritic injury) or an exogenous (circulating) factor.

Neurofibrillary Tangles

Alzheimer's original description (Wilkins and Brody, 1969) demonstrates his remarkable powers of observation:

In sections prepared with the Bielschowsky silver method, remarkable changes in the neurofibrils appeared. In the interior of a cell that otherwise appeared normal, one or several fibrils stood out due to their extraordinary thickness and impregnability. At a later stage, many fibrils appeared, situated side by side and altered in the same way. Then they merged into dense bundles and reached the surface of the cell. Finally, the nucleus and the cell disintegrated and only a dense bundle of fibrils indicated the site where a ganglion cell had been.

Nothing was added to this concept of NF for 55 years.

Terry (1963) and Kidd (1963) presented ultrastructural evidence that NF were composed of twisted linear structures 240 Å thick at their nontwisted part. Terry (1963) and later Hirano et al. (1968) considered these to be twisted tubules, hence analogous to microtubules. Kidd (1968) on the other hand believed that these were twisted helical filaments that were similar to 100-Å-thick neurofilaments. Recently Wisniewski et al. (1976) showed that the tangles are composed of bifilar helices made up of 130-Å filaments.

To anyone except a cell biologist these designations must appear to represent trivia. But they have relevance to neuronal pathophysiology and an understanding of their nature and function seems necessary. The neuron (and probably most cells) manufactures three fibrillar proteins, actin, tubulin, and neurofilament protein, probably at the centriole region of the cell. While the basic protein subunit is similar (50,000–65,000 mol. wt.), differences in solubility, amino acid composition and electrophoretic migration clearly distinguish each as a separate entity, and these are not considered to be interchangeable (DeBrabander et al., 1975).

Actin is the principal component of microfilaments, which are contractile structures about 60 Å thick. They are believed to control the shape of the cell and seem particularly important in axon extension. Tubulin is actually a dimer of protein subunits, 53,000 and 56,000 mol. wt. (Feit et al., 1971) and is the major component of neurotubules (microtubules). Neurotubules are hollow structures 240 Å in thickness. While they are noncontractile they appear to form a structural unit upon which intracellular transport occurs. Directed transport is possible by continual dispersion and reassembly of these structures. Neurofilaments are linear structures, 100 Å in diameter and composed of subunits that are 68,000 mol. wt. (Schlaepfer, 1977). The function of this protein is not known at this time. The important aspect of these proteins is that after their formation in the cell body, they move distally within the axon. This seems to occur within the slow component of axoplasmic movement at a rate of 1 mm per day (Hoffman and Lasek, 1975).

A most important aspect of these protein subunits is their ability to exist either as a structured organelle or as dispersed subunits in the cytoplasm. The chemical character of the subunit undoubtedly controls the linkage and ultimate form of the structure (Borisy and Olmstead, 1972). However the aggregation and dispersion of the subunits are profoundly affected by ionic conditions of the cytoplasm and by certain agents such as colchicine and vinblastine (Weisenberg and Timasheff, 1970).

The evolution of neurofibrillary pathology can now be presented as two distinct possible sequences. The primary event can be an abnormality of fibrous protein synthesis or of a cell environment that affects subunit aggregation. The resulting abnormal filaments affect cytoplasmic flow particularly in axons and dendrites to cause dilation of these neurites and degeneration of synaptic terminals. The neurites and synapses degenerate and form the origin of a senile plaque. There are three major problems with this concept. (1) The identification of abnormal fibrous protein in AD (Iqbal et al., 1975) remains controversial and must be clarified. (2) The focal aggregates of thickened neurites are probably derived from many cells quite distant from the cell body. It is very difficult to explain this localized change on the basis of altered cytoplasmic transport beginning in the cell body. (3) A functional relationship between neurofilaments and cytoplasmic transport has not been proven. In other words these proteins are partaking in transport but they are probably not controlling it.

The alternative concept is that the proliferation of filamentous structures represents a neuronal response to the injury of distant axons and dendrites manifested as thickened neurites. A most likely initial event would involve an exogenous agent affecting distal nerve fibers in such a way to produce a block of axon flow. In experimental animals this can occur secondary to nerve compression (Weiss, 1961) or by a dispersion of microtubules. Microtubules can be disrupted by a variety of experimental circumstances including elevation of Ca^{2+} (Schlaepfer and Bunge, 1975) and the use of mitotic spindle inhibitors such as vincristine (Schlaepfer, 1971). Increased filament aggregates have been observed repeatedly following destruction of microtubules not only in neurons (Wisniewski et al., 1964) but also in muscle (Ishikawa et al., 1968). This has been considered to represent either reconversion of tubulin subunits or an aggregation of dispersed filamentous protein, but DeBrabander et al. (1975) have shown that this is due to new protein synthesis. This proliferation of filaments in the neuron is a well-recognized response to distant injury and has been noted after axon section (Pannese, 1963) and in vincristine neuropathy (Shelanski et al., 1969).

A secondary evolution of NF is more consistent with the idea that SP and NF are related manifestations of the same problem. In this concept the SP, particularly the neuritic plaque, would be the initial lesion. Neurite injury at the terminal part of their anatomy would not be expected to elicit the same response as major axon section, so cumulative injury seems necessary to induce the cell body reaction. The greater frequency of plaques versus tangles in nondemented people (Tomlinson et al., 1968) and the widespread occurrence of NF in the greater devastation of AD before 65 would be in agreement with this proposal. Perhaps the most important aspect of this viewpoint is that NF would not be an indicator of imminent cell destruction. If the injury is repaired as it is in peripheral nerve axon section, the cell body could return to normal. This may also explain why Ball (1977) found that the severity of NF in the posterior hippocampus is proportionally more severe in dementia than would be anticipated by the neuronal loss.

There are numerous diseases of the brain in which NF are found in the absence of SP. Among others, these include the Parkinson-dementia complex of Guam (Hirano et al., 1961), progressive supranuclear palsy (Steele et al., 1964), and boxer brains (Corsellis et al., 1973). In these circumstances, a primary dysfunction of fibril metabolism must be considered quite possible. Indeed the variations of neurofibrillary pathology that are demonstrable by means of electron microscopy (Wisniewski et al., 1970a) should indicate that they have a multivariate etiology. By way of contrast with the usual 240-Å twisted structures, 100-Å straight filaments occur in bundles in supranuclear palsy (Tellez-Nagel and Wisniewski, H.M., 1973) twisted and straight 100–150-Å filaments arranged as a round body are seen in Pick's disease (Brion, 1973; Schrochet et al., 1968), and 60–100-Å filaments aggregate with electron dense bodies to form sheets in Hirano bodies, which were described originally in the Parkinsonism-dementia complex of Guam (Hirano et al., 1961). At the present time we do not know whether these variations are due to peculiarities of protein synthesis or to cell environment but one or the other would appear to be responsible for them. As a final comment, we must add that these peculiar fibrous proteins apparently have little potential (except in Pick's disease) to be an endogenous substrate for amyloid synthesis.

Creutzfeldt-Jakob Disease

The pathologic criteria for CJD appear to be quite distinctive and they would seem to preclude any confusion regarding classification or nomenclature. Yet we find, in addition to CJD, such terminology as Jakob-Creutzfeldt disease, Heidenhain's syndrome, subacute sclerosing encephalopathy, "classic" Jakob-Creutzfeldt disease, and many more. The reason for this diversity lies in the fact that the "classic" triad of status spongsiosis, neuronal destruction, and severe gliosis is not present in every case of subacute dementia. The spongy state, which is accepted to be a distinctive change, was not present in Creutzfeldt's original case and indeed it occurred only in the fifth case reported by Jakob between 1921 and 1923 (Kirschbaum, 1968). The early history of this entity seems worth of review.

Alfons Jakob was the unquestioned originator of the entity we know as Creutzfeldt-Jakob disease (Hassin, 1953; Kirschbaum, 1968). As a result of earlier studies on tract degeneration, he became interested in spastic pseudosclerosis. Soon he had collected five cases in which a variety of motor problems were associated with a rapidly progressive dementia. He believed these cases were distinguishable from amyotrophic lateral sclerosis and muscle atrophies. In his search of the literature he decided that a case report published by Creutzfeldt in 1920 was similar to his cases. This selection was inopportune because it led to an eponymic debate; should the organizer or a fortuitous author receive top billing? Irrespective of a Creutzfeldt-Jakob or Jakob-Creutzfeldt title, these cases had a dramatic clinical course but the pathologic correlates were comparatively subtle. (1) There was no significant brain atrophy. (2) There were no distinctive morphologic changes in neurons. (3) A distinct fibrous gliosis was not present despite clusters of hypertrophied protoplasmic astrocytes. The fifth case of Jakob was clearly different:

> The entire cortex was the site of most severe alterations. Many neurons presented shrunken, sclerotic, swollen, inflated, and vacuolated forms of degeneration accompanied by astrocytic proliferations. The appearance of the larger neurons of the fifth layer was suggestive of axonal degeneration. The three lower cortical laminae showed most severe disturbances, single losses of neurons, aggregated areolar neuronal depletion among abundant hypertrophic protoplasmic and also fibrous astrocytes.

Next followed 2 case reports by Kirschbaum, both with status spongiosis, and 3 by Heidenhain, 2 of which had status spongiosis. Heidenhain's cases all had visual agnosia with severe occipital lobe involvement and he proposed that his cases and Kirschbaum's were different from those of Creutzfeldt and Jakob because of the visual-occipital disease rather than the spongiosis. This "occipito-parietal agnostic-visual and dyskinetic syndrome" was noted also by Meyer in 1929, who called it "Heidenhain's syndrome" and the sponginess was not mentioned as a unique pathologic change. Indeed nosologic significance was not attributed to the severe vacuolation until 1954, when Jones and Nevin felt that it characterized their 2 cases. In 1959 Alema and Bignami used occipital involvement and sponginess to separate their two examples of subacute dementia. In 1960 Nevin et al. formalized status spongiosis as a determinant in their concept of "subacute spongiform encephalopathy". The other (nonspongiform) cases were called "classic" Jakob-Creutzfeldt disease.

At this point a very strange evolution of thought occurred. The vascular etiology of subacute spongiform encephalopathy proposed by Nevin et al. was not generally accepted but the spongy change was proclaimed as a uniform change of subacute dementia (Siedler and Malamud, 1963). From this time on, CJD became equated with status spongiosis and intense gliosis. The real question should not be whether Creutzfeldt or Jakob is preeminent but why Nevin is not only ignored as an originator of spongiform encephalopathy but even scorned for his concept of vascular etiology. The whole problem was resolved by the transmission of encephalopathy to a chimpanzee (Gibbs et al., 1968). Transmissible viral dementia (TVD) was established and the animal disease was characterized by status spongiosis.

TVD is characterized uniformly by a spongiform encephalopathy which involves both neurons and astrocytes (Lampert et al., 1971). The vacuolation is due to a low-density enlargement of neuronal cell bodies, axons, dendrites, and synapses with similar changes in astrocytes but with no evident widening of extracellular spaces. These swellings apparently are the result of an altered cell membrane, and can be identified in electron micrographs as discontinuities accompanied by curling of the disjoined parts. The same abnormality has been described in experimental scrapie, and in experimental kuru (Lampert et al., 1972). Some alteration of cell membrane permeability is very compatible with the evolution of cellular swelling.

This appeared to duplicate the ultrastructural features of CJD in brain biopsies (Gonatas et al., 1965; Kidd, 1967; Bignami and Forno, 1970; Foncin, 1967). These studies established a new structural correlate to neuronal disease. Diffuse neuron swelling has always been recognized as an acute reaction to various injuries (anoxia, hypoglycemia, CO poisoning). However in CJD there was focal swelling in cell bodies in the form of membrane-bound sacs (Gonatas et al., 1965; Kidd, 1967) or in localized segments of preterminal axons or presynaptic nerve endings (Bignami and Forno, 1970). While these changes suggested an abnormal membrane permeability no ruptures like those found by Lambert in TVD were described in the human biopsy studies. The astrocytic swelling apparently indicates a primary abnormality of these cells. This may be important in the development of the intense fibrous gliosis but its role in neuronal dysfunction is unclear at this time.

The pathology of CJD also includes plaquelike masses that contain amyloid but may or may not be surrounded by thickened neurites (Adams et al., 1974). Electron microscopy (Chou and Martin, 1971; Hirano et al., 1972) confirmed the amyloid nature of the plaques in both instances with no explanation regarding the presence or absence of neurites. No plaques have been reported in TVD, but, as noted earlier, plaques with amyloid and abnormal neurites have been noted in scrapie-infected mice (Wisniewski et al., 1976).

The etiologic agent of slow virus encephalopathy has not been identified, but in scrapie, this agent has been considered to be composed of a single strand of DNA surrounded by a polysaccharide coat (Adams, 1973). Narang (1975) has identified 90-Å particles in CJD biopsies, which is similar to much more convincing arrays of similar particles in scrapie-infected sheep and rodent brain (Narang, 1974). These particles also appear to have a polysaccharide coat stainable by ruthenium red (Narang, 1974a). Unfortunately it has not been possible to isolate these particles. Of considerable interest is their occurrence in dendrites and distal axons including synaptic endings. Vacuolation of dendrites with cell membrane abnormality has been emphasized by Lampert et al. (1975) in virus encephalopathy. No NF have been demonstrated in TVD.

The various histochemical and biochemical assays in CJD have revealed decreased oxidative enzyme activity (Friede and DeJong, 1965; Robinson, 1969) and increased acid phosphatase activity (Friede and DeJong, 1967; Torack, 1969). Biochemical assays have generally revealed decreased levels of various components most consistent with neuronal destruction (Suzuki, 1966; Bass et al., 1974). A prominent loss of ganglioside has been noted in both studies and suggests a change in cell membranes. Virus inactivation by membrane-disrupting substances (Gibbs and Gajdusek, 1974) indicates an association of virus with these membranes. It is tempting to propose a realtionship between the polysaccharide coat of the theorized organism (Adams, 1973) and the sialic acid component of the cell membrane. Lampert et al. (1975a) has shown recently that measles virus can strip off these cell membrane components as it attacks the cell. This could be an explanation of the cell swelling.

In summary a spongiform subacute encephalopathy has been shown to be transmissible to experimental animals and is compatible with a slow virus etiology despite the lack of identification of this agent. Subacute dementia without a spongiform change has not been used for transmission experiments. Focal swelling of neurons and astrocytes appears to be a distinctive cellular change and may be the result of an action by the infectious agent upon the cell membrane. This action constitutes the best evidence that this agent has been transmitted.

Other Pathologic Correlates

Aluminum

The association of aluminum with AD originated when aluminum was shown to cause NF in rabbits (Klatzo et al., 1965). The significance of this finding was considered to be of great importance since it constituted the first experimental induction of NF and of any of the morphologic correlates of AD. Terry and Pena (1965) studied these tangles by means of electron microscopy and showed that they were composed of 100-Å straight filaments. The neurotoxicity of aluminum was demonstrated more definitively by its presence in neurons 10 weeks after an intracerebral injection and, after 2 years, most of the neurons were labeled with aluminum (Stercova, 1966). The etiologic significance of aluminum for AD appeared enhanced when Wisniewski and Terry (1968) succeeded in producing neuritic plaques with aluminum. It seemed confirmed by the presence of elevated aluminum levels in the cortex of AD (Crapper et al., 1973) and by the demonstration of memory loss and abnormal behavior in cats injected with aluminum (Crapper and Dalton, 1973).

Since that time, much inconsistency has occurred in experiments with aluminum. Several authors (Klatzo et al., 1965; Stercova, 1966) remarked quite clearly that aluminum diffused extensively through the brain and frequently the injection site was not detectable. Apparently the site of injection did not change the distribution of the tangles because of this diffusibility. But Harris (1973) using Amphojel observed a local granuloma even after 5.5 years and no neuronal involvement. Either the species (monkey) or the type of aluminum (Amphojel) was the cause of this discrepancy. Aluminum in neurons was identified in neurons by Stercova but only after 10 weeks whereas De Boni et al. (1974) found neuronal involvement after 6 h. Perhaps most interesting was the finding that neuronal involvement was not uniform, predominantly affecting the brain stem and spinal cord (Wisniewski et al., 1967) with minimal cortical change. Yet Stercova noted diffuse cortical involvement after 2 years and Harris, none. Within neurons Stercova described cytoplasmic granules but according to De Boni et al. the aluminum was bound to nuclear chromatin.

The studies of human material reveal similar inconsistencies. Crapper et al. (1973) found the highest cortical levels in mesial, frontal, and temporal areas but noted a wide range in the quantity of this deposit even at these sites. However early studies of neuronal enriched fractions have revealed no detectable aluminum (Wisniewski, 1975), and Duckett and Galle (1976), using an electron probe, have reported that the aluminum was in SP. There have been two human cases that appeared to represent true aluminum encephalopathy and neither case had NF (McLaughlin et al., 1962; Lapresle et al., 1975). The first was a 47-year-old aluminum worker whose brain had 17 times the normal content of aluminum with no abnormal morphology (AD is mentioned specifically) and no clinical dementia (McLaughlin et al., 1962). The other case was a 37-year-old alcoholic with no history of aluminum exposure. He had a recurrent and progressive neurologic syndrome reminiscent of multiple sclerosis. Autopsy revealed many foci of white-matter demyelination with a core of inorganic material chiefly composed of aluminum phosphate (Lapresle et al., 1973).

Despite these variable findings, the potential for aluminum as en etiological agent for Alzheimer's disease remains because of its proven neurotoxicity that appears to stimulate basic protein synthesis (Exss and Summer, 1973). Berlyne et al. (1972) have shown that aluminum crosses the blood-brain barrier so a brain effect due to an exogenous source seems possible. The neuronal selectivity of aluminum toxicity indicates that specific neurological syndromes are possible. Widespread use of aluminum constitutes a ready source of contamination but a major difficulty seems to be the apparent lack of dementia among aluminum workers (McLaughlin et al., 1962).

Lipofuscin

In contrast to its importance in aging, lipofuscin has never been considered to be an essential aspect of Alzheimer's disease. Prominent pigmentation of neurons has been a constant finding of intact neurons but these nerve cells are considered to be old and not sick. The controversy regarding the significance of lipofuscin accrues primarily because it lacks a defined pathogenicity. Its increase in aging is unquestioned but no one has demonstrated that this is a forerunner of neuronal death. Lipofuscin appears early in the life of vital cells (cranial nerve nuclei, anterior horn cells) and it is prominent in the inferior olive where recent studies have shown no neuron loss with age (Monagle and Brody, 1974).

As a neuronal modification of a lysosome, the lipofuscin body must be considered to have a potential role in neuronal degeneration. The increased acid phosphatase in CJD has been shown to be in a lipofuscin body (Torack, 1969) and is believed to be related to an increased activity of this degradative pathway (Torack, 1971). Abnormal lipofuscin has been demonstrated in an unusual case of progressive dementia (Torack, 1966) and it has been considered to reflect altered protein metabolism. Recently similar lipofuscin has been reported in Huntington's chorea (Tellez-Nagel, 1973) in which a disorder of histone metabolism is also suspected (Iqbal et al., 1974). There is no evidence to suggest that a primary dysfunction of a lipofuscin body is the cause of Alzheimer's disease.

Granulovacuolar Degeneration

The ultrastructure of granulovacuolar degeneration has been demonstrated quite capably by Hirano et al. (1968). It is a membrane bound cytoplasmic body containing an irregular electron dense core surrounded by electron lucent material. The function of this body in neuronal degeneration is not affected by this information, it is just a puzzling now as it was prior to electron microscopy.

Pathogenetic Implications of Pathology

No etiological agents have been characterized completely by the new technology even in CJD where a slow virus etiology seems certain. However considerably less specific data about the nature of the cause or causes of dementia have been determined. The spongiform degeneration in CJD is a distinctive type of neuronal destruction involving cell membranes which is transmitted by a slow virus. This degree of status spongiosis is not characteristic of typical Alzheimer's disease, so a slow viral etiology is not supported by these findings. However the occurrence of senile plaques in scrapie mice indicates that an infectious etiology cannot be discounted. Two different types of senile plaques are suggested. The neuritic plaque seems to have local evolution and is compatible with aluminum intoxication or an endognous brain disorder such as aging. A perivascular amyloid plaque has been related to congophilic angiopathy and an exogenous etiological agent in the circulation. This agent is age related. It can be transferred hereditarily and in mice, it is either associated with or identical to the scrapie agent.

Neurofibrillary tangles generally seem to represent a reactive change to peripheral neurite injury affecting axoplasmic movement. Primary protein dysmetabolism remains a possibility in unusual forms of human dementia when these lesions are unassociated with senile plaques. Aluminum has been shown to have definite neurotoxicity and the capability to induce neurofibrillary tangles in experimental animals. The confusing array of reports involving aluminum deposition in human disease render its association with Alzheimer's disease inconclusive. Nevertheless its potential as a cause of Alzheimer's disease remains positive. Lipofuscin and granulovacuolar degeneration are indeterminent factors in the evolution of Alzheimer's disease since their pathogenicity has not been demonstrated.

References

Adams, D.H. (1973): Nucleic acids and slow virus infections. Biochem. Soc. Symp. 540 Meeting 1, 1061–1064

Adams, H., Beck, E., Shenkin, A.M. (1974): Creutzfeldt-Jakob disease: Further similarities with Kuru. J. Neurol. Neurosurg. Psychiatry 37, 195–200

Alema, G., Bignami, A. (1959): Polioencephalopatia degenerative subacuta del presenio con stuppore acinetico e rigidita decorticata con mioclonie. Rio Sper. Freniat. 83 (Suppl. 4), 1491

Alzheimer, A. (1904): Histologische Studien zur Differentialdiagnose der progressiven Paralyse. Nissl's Arbeiten 1, 18

Austin, J.H., Rinehart, R., Williamson, T., Burcar, P., Russ, K., Nikaido, T., LaFrance, M. (1973): Studies in aging of the brain. III. Silicon levels in postmortem tissues and body fluids. Prog. Brain Res. 40, 486–495

Ball, M.J. (1976): Neurofibrillary tangles and the pathogenesis of dementia: A quantitative study. Neuropathol. Appl. Neurobiol. 2, 395–410

Bass, N.H., Hess, H.H., Pope, A. (1974): Altered cell membranes in Creutzfeldt-Jakob disease. Arch. Neurol. 31, 174–182

Berlyne, G.M., Ben Ari, J., Knopf, E., Yagil, R., Weinberger, G., Danovitch, G.M. (1972): Aluminum toxicity in rats. Lancet 2, 564–567

Bignami, A., Forno, L.S. (1970): Status spongiosis in Jakob-Creutzfeldt disease. Electron microscopic study of a cortical biopsy. Brain 93, 89–94

Blessed, G., Tomlinson, B.E., Roth, M. (1968): The association between quantitative measures of dementia and of senile change in the cerebral grey matter of elderly subjects. Br. J. Psychiatry 114, 797–811

Borisy, G.G., Olmstead, J.B. (1972): Nucleated assembly of microtubules in porcine brain extracts. Science 177, 1196–1197

Brion, S., Mikol, J., Psimaras, A. (1973): Recent findings in Pick's disease. In: Progress in Neuropathology. Zimmerman, H.M. (ed.). New York: Grune and Stratton, pp. 421–451

Chou, S.M., Martin, J.D. (1971): Kuru plaques in a case of Creutzfeldt-Jakob disease. Acta Neuropathol. 17, 150–155

Cohen, A.S., Calkins, E. (1959): Electron microscopic observations on a fibrous component in amyloid of diverse origins. Nature 183, 1202–1203

Corsellis, J.A.N., Brierly, J.B. (1954): An unusual type of presenile dementia. Brain 77, 571–587

Corsellis, J.A.N., Bruton, C.H., Freeman-Browne, D. (1973): The aftermath of boxing. Psychol. Med. 3, 270–303

Crapper, D.R., Dalton, A.J. (1973): Alterations in short term retention, conditioned avoidance response acquisition and motivation following aluminum induced neurofibrillary degeneration. Physiol. Behav. 10, 925–933

Crapper, D.R., Krishnan, S.S., Dalton, A.J. (1973): Brain aluminum distribution in Alzheimer's disease and experimental neurofibrillary degeneration. Science 180, 511–513

DeBoni, Scott, J.W., Crapper, D.R. (1974): Intracellular aluminum binding; a histochemical study. Histochemie 40, 31–37

DeBrabander, M., Aerts, F., Van DeVere, R., Borgers, M. (1975): Evidence against interconversion of microtubules and filaments. Nature 253, 119–120

Divry, P. (1927): Etude histochimique des plaques séniles. J. Belge Neurol. 27, 643–657

Divry, P. (1952): La pathochimie générale et cellulaire des processus séniles et préséniles. Proc. 1st Int. Cong. Neuropathol. 2, 313–345

Duckett, S., Galle, P. (1976): Mise en évidence de l'aluminum dans les plaques séniles de la maladie d'Alzheimer: étude à la microsonde de Castaing. C.R. Acad. Sci. [D] (Paris) 282, 393–395

Exss, R.E., Summer, G.K. (1973): Basic proteins in neurons containing fibrillary deposits. Brain Res. 49, 151–164

Feit, H., Slusarch, L., Shelanski, M.L. (1971): Heterogeneity of tubulin subunits. Proc. Natl. Acad. Sci. 68, 2028–2031

Ferraro, A. (1931): The origin and formation of senile plaques. Arch. Neurol. Psychiatry 25, 1042–1062

Fischer, O. (1910): Die presbyophrene Demenz, deren anatomische Grundlage und klinische Abgrenzung. Z. Neurol. Psychiatr. 3, 371–471

Foncin, J.F. (1967): Electron microscopic observations in Creutzfeldt-Jakob disease. Acta Neuropathol. (Suppl.) III, 171–177

Friede, R.L., DeJong, R.N. (1964): Neuronal enzymatic failure in Creutzfeldt-Jakob disease. Arch. Neurol. 10, 181–195

Friede, R.L. (1965): Enzyme histochemical studies of senile plaques. J. Neuropathol. Exp. Neurol. 24, 477–491

Fuller, S. (1911): A study of the miliary plaques found in brains of the aged. Am. J. Ins. 68, 147–217

Gerhard, L., Bergener, M., Homayan, S. (1972): Angiopathie bei Alzheimerscher Krankheit. Z. Neurol. 201, 43–61

Gibbs, C.J., Jr., Gajdusek, D.C., Asher, D.M., Alpers, M.P. (1968): Creutzfeldt-Jakob disease (spongiform encephalophathy): Transmission to the chimpanzee. Science 161, 388–389

Gibbs, C.J., Jr., Gajdusek, D.C. (1974): Cell-virus interactions in slow infections of the nervous system. In: The Neurosciences. Third Study Probram. Schmitt, F.O., Worden, F.G. (eds.). Cambridge: MIT Press

Glenner, G.G., Page, D., Isersky, C., Harada, M., Cuatrecases, P., Eanes, E.D., DeLellis, R.A., Bladen, H.A., Keiser, H.R. (1971): Murine amyloid fibril protein: Isolation, purification and characterization. J. Histochem. Cytochem. 19, 16–28

Glenner, G.G., Terry, W.D., Isersky, C. (1973): Amyloidosis: Its nature and pathogenesis. Semin. Hematol. 10, 65–86

Goldman, R.D. (1971): The role of three cytoplasmic fibers in BHK-21 cell motility. I. Microtubules and the effects of colchicine. J. Cell Biol. 51, 752–762

Gonatas, N.K., Terry, R.D., Weiss, M. (1965): Electron microscopical study in two cases of Jakob-Creutzfeldt disease. J. Neuropathol. Exp. Neurol. 24, 575–598

Gonatas, N., Anderson, W., Evangelista, I. (1967): The contribution of altered synapses in the senile plaque: An electron microscopic study in Alzheimer dementia. J. Neuropathol. Exp. Neurol. 26, 25–39

Harris, A.B. (1973): Ultrastructure and histochemistry of alumina in cortex. Exp. Neurol. 38, 33–63

Hassin, G. (1953): Alfons Maria Jakob. In: Founders of Neurology. Haymaker, W. (ed.). Springfield: Thomas

Hirano, A., Malamud, N., Kurland, L.T. (1961): Parkinsonism-dementia complex, an endemic disease on the island of Guam. 2. Pathological features. Brain 84, 662–679

Hirano, A., Dembither, H.M., Jurland, L.T., Zimmerman, H.M. (1968): The fine structure of some intraganglionic alterations. J. Neuropathol. Exp. Neurol. 27, 167–182

Hirano, A., Ghatak, N.R., Johnson, A.B., Partnow, M.J., Gomori, A.J. (1972): Argentophilic plaques in Creutzfeldt-Jakob disease. Arch. Neurol. 26, 530–542

Hoffman, P.N., Lasek, R.J. (1975): The slow component of axonal transport. J. Cell. Biol. 66, 351–366

Hollander, D., Strich, S.J. (1968): Atypical Alzheimer's disease with congophilic angiopathy presenting with dementia of acute onset. In: Alzheimer's Disease and Related Conditions. Wolstenholme, G.E.W., O'Connor, M. (eds.). London: Churchill, pp. 105–135

Iqbal, K., Tellez-Nagel, I., Grundke-Iqbal (1974): Protein abnormalities in Huntington's chorea. Brain Res. 76, 178–184

Iqbal, K., Wisniewski, H.M., Grundke, Iqbal, I., Korthals, J.K., Terry, R.D. (1975): Chemical pathology of neurofibrils. Neurofibrillary tangles of Alzheimer's presenile-senile dementia. J. Histochem. Cytochem. 23, 563–569

Ishikawa, H., Bischoff, R., Holtzer, H. (1968): Mitosis and intermediate sized filaments in developing skeletal muscle, J. Cell. Biol. 38, 538–555

Jellinger, K. (1977): Cerebrovascular amyloidosis with cerebral hemorrhage. J. Neurol. 214, 195–206

Jervis, G.A., Soltz, S.E. (1936): Alzheimer's disease – the so called juvenile type. Am. J. Psychiatry 93, 39–56

Johnson, A.B., Blum, N.R. (1970): Nucleoside phosphatase activities associated with the tangles and plaques of Alzheimer's disease. A histochemical study of natural and experimental neurofibrillary tangles. J. Neuropathol. Exp. Neurol. 29, 463–478

Jones, D.P., Nevin (1954): Rapidly progressive cerebral degeneration (subacute vascular encephalopathy) with mental disorder, focal disturbances, and myoclonic epilepsy. J. Neurol. Neurosurg. Psychiatry 17, 148–159

Josephy, H. (1949): Acid phosphatase in the senile brain. Arch. Neurol. Psychiatry 61, 164–169

Kidd, M. (1963): Paired helical filaments in electron microscopy of Alzheimer's disease. Nature 197, 192–193

Kidd, M. (1964): Alzheimer's disease – an electron microscopical study. Brain 87, 307–320

Kidd, M. (1967): Some electron microscopical observations on status spongiosis. Acta Neuropathol. (Suppl.) III, 137–144

98

Kirschbaum, W.R. (1968): Jakob-Creutzfeldt Disease. New York; Elsevier

Klatzo, I., Wisniewski, H., Streicher, E. (1965): Experimental production of neurofibrillary degeneration. J. Neuropathol. Exp. Neurol. 24, 187–199

Krigman, M.R., Feldman, R.G., Bensch, K. (1965): Alzheimer's presenile dementia. Lab. Invest. 14, 381–396

Lampert, P.W., Gajdusek, D.C., Gibbs, C.J., Jr. (1971): Experimental spongiform encephalopathy (Creutzfeldt-Jakob disease) in chimpanzees. J. Neuropathol. Exp. Neurol. 30, 20–32

Lampert, P.W., Gajdusek, D.C., Gibbs, C.J., Jr. (1972): Subacute spongiform virus encephalopathies. Am. J. Pathol. 68, 626–646

Lampert, P.W., Gajdusek, D.C., Gibbs, C.J., Jr. (1975a): Pathology of dendrites in subacute spongiform virus encephalopathies. Adv. Neurol. 12, 465–470

Lampert, P.W., Joseph, B.S., Oldstone, M.B.A. (1975): Antibody-induced capping of measles virus antigens on plasma membrane studied by electron microscopy. J. Virol. 15, 1248–1255

Lapresle, J., Duckett, S., Galle, P., Cartier, L. (1975): Documents cliniques, anatomiques et biophysiques dans une encéphalopathie avec présence de dépôts d'aluminum. C.R. Soc. Biol. (Paris) 169, 282–287

Ley, R. (1922): Etude anatomique sur la sénilité. In: Livre Jubilaire de la Société Belge de Neurologie

Lowenberg, K. (1928): Zur Frage der elektiven Gefäßerkrankung. J. Psychol. Neurol. 36, 81–86

Luers, T. (1947): Über die familiäre juvenile Form der Alzheimerschen Krankheit mit neurologischen Herderscheinungen. Arch. Psychiatr. Nervenkr. 179, 132–145

MacKeown, E.F. (1965): Pathology of the Aged. London: Butterworths

Mandybur, T.I. (1975): The incidence of cerebral amyloid angiopathy in Alzheimer's disease. Neurology 25, 120–126

McLaughlin, A.I.G., Kazantzis, G., King, E., Teare, D., Porter, R.J., Owen, R. (1962): Pulmonary fibrosis and encephalopathy associated with the inhalation of aluminum dust. Br. J. Ind. Med. 19, 253–263

Meyer, A. (1929): Über eine der amyotrophischen Lateralsklerose nahestehende Erkrankung mit psychischen Störungen. Z. Neurol. Psychiatr. 1212, 107–138

Morek, F., Wildi, E. (1952): General and cellular pathochemistry of senile and presenile alterations of the brain. Proc. 1st Int. Cong. Neuropathol. 2, 347–374

Morimatsu, M., Hirai, S., Muramatsu, A., Yosikawa, M. (1975): Senile degenerative brain lesions and dementia. J. Am. Geriatr. Soc. 23, 390–406

Narang, H.K. (1974): An electron microscopic study of the scrapie mouse and rat: Further observations on virus-like particles with ruthenium red and lanthanum nitrate as a possible trace and negative stain. Neurobiol. 4, 349–363

Narang, H.K. (1974a): An electron microscopic study of natural scrapie sheep brain: Further observations on virus-like particles and paramyxovirus-like tubules. Acta Neuropathol. 28, 317–329

Narang, H.K. (1975): Virus like particles in Creutzfeldt-Jakob biopsy material. Acta Neuropathol. 32, 163–168

Neumann, M. (1960): Combined amyloid vascular changes and argyrophilic plaques in the central nervous system. J. Neuropathol. Exp. Neurol. 19, 370–382

Nevin, S., McMenemey, W.H., Behrman, S., Jones, D.P. (1960): Subacute spongiform encephalopathy – A subacute form of encephalopathy attributable to vascular dysfunction (spongiform cerebral atrophy). Brain 83, 519–564

Nikaido, T., Austin, J., Rinehart, R., Trueb, L., Hutchinson, J., Stukenbrok, H., Miles, B. (1971): Studies in aging of the brain. I. Isolation and preliminary characterization of Alzheimer plaques and cores. Arch. Neurol. 25, 198–211

Pannese, E. (1963): Investigations on the ultrastructural changes of the spinal ganglion neurons in the course of axon regeneration and cell hypertrophy. Z. Zellforsch. 60, 711–740

Redlich, E. (1898): Über miliare Sklerose der Hirnrinde bei seniler Atrophie. Jahrb. Psychiatr. Neurol. 17, 208–216

Robinson, N. (1969): Creutzfeldt-Jakob's disease: A histochemical study. Brain 92, 581–588

Schlaepfer, W.W. (1971): Vincristine-induced axonal alterations in rat peripheral nerve. J. Neuropathol. Exp. Neurol. 30, 488–505

Schlaepfer, W.W., Bunge, R.P. (1973): Effects of calcium on concentration on the degeneration of amputated axons in tissue culture. J. Cell. Biol. 59, 456–470

Schlaepfer, W.W. (1977): Immunological and ultrastructural studies of neurofilaments isolated from rat peripheral nerve. J. Cell. Biol. 74, 226–240

Schlote, W. (1965): Die amyloide Natur der kongophilen drüsigen Entartung der Hirnarterien (Scholz) im Senium. Acta Neuropathol. 4, 449–468

Schrochet, S.S., Lampert, P.W., Lindenberg, R. (1968): Fine structure of the Pick and Hirano bodies in a case of Pick's disease. Acta Neuropathol. 11, 330–337

Schwartz, P. (1970): Amyloidosis: Cause and Manifestations of Senile Deterioration. Springfield: C.C. Thomas

Seitelberger, F. (1974): Dementia following non-arteriosclerotic vascular processes of the CNS. In: Cerebral Vascular Disease. Meyer, J.S., Lechman, H., Reivich, M., Eichhorn, O. (eds.). St. Louis: C.V. Mosvy, pp. 200–206

Shelanski, M.L., Wisniewski, H.M. (1969): Neurofibrillary degeneration. Arch. Neurol. 20, 199–206

Scholz, W. (1938): Studien zur Pathologie der Hirngefäße. II. Die drüsige Entartung der Hirnarterien und Kapillaren. Z. Neurol. Psychiatr. 162, 694–715

Siedler, H., Malamud, N. (1963): Creutzfeldt-Jakob disease. J. Neuropathol. Exp. Neurol. 22, 381–402

Simchowicz, T. (1910): Histologische Studien über die senile Demenz. Nissl's Arbeiten 4, 267

Stercova, A. (1966): Dynamics of neurohistopathological changes in an epileptogenic focus produced by alumina in the rat. In: Comparative and Cellular Pathophysiology of Epilepsy. Servit, Z. (ed.). New York: Excerpta Med., pp. 247–255

Steele, J.C. (1972): Progressive supra nuclear palsy. Brain 95, 693–704

Suzuki, F., Katzman, R., Korey, S. (1965): Chemical studies of Alzheimer's disease. J. Neuropathol. Exp. Neurol. 14, 211–222

Suzuki, F., Chen, G. (1966): Chemical studies on Jakob-Creutzfeldt disease. J. Neuropathol. Exp. Neurol. 25, 396–408

Suzuki, F., Terry, R.D. (1967): Fine structural localization of acid phosphatase in senile plaques in Alzheimer's presenile dementia. Acta Neuropathol. 8, 276–284

Tellez-Nagel, I., Kohnson, A.B., Terry, R.D. (1973): Ultrastructural and histochemical study of cerebral biopsies in Huntington's chorea. Adv. Neurol. 1, 387–398

Tellez-Nagel, I., Wisniewski, H.M. (1973): Ultrastructure of neurofibrillary tangles in Steele-Richardson-Olszewski syndrome. Arch. Neurol. 29, 324–327

Terry, R.D. (1963): The fine structure of neurofibrillary tangles in Alzheimer's disease. J. Neuropathol. Exp. Neurol. 22, 629–634

Terry, R.D., Gonatas, N.K., Weiss, M. (1964): Ultrastructural studies in Alzheimer's presenile dementia. Am. J. Pathol. 44, 269–297

Tomlinson, B.E., Blessed, G., Roth, M. (1968): Observations on the brains of non-demented old people. J. Neurol. Sci. 7, 331–356

Tomlinson, B.E., Blessed, G., Roth, M. (1970): Observations on the brains of demented old people. J. Neurol. Sci. 11, 205

Tomlinson, B.E. (1977): Morphological changes and dementia in old age. In: Aging and Dementia. Smith, W.L., Kinsbourne, M. (eds.). New York: Spectrum, pp. 25–86

Torack, R.M. (1969): Ultrastructural and histochemical studies of cortical biopsies in subacute dementia. Acta Neuropathol. 13, 43–55

Torack, R.M. (1971): Studies in the pathology of dementia. In: Dementia, The Failing Brain. Wells, C. (ed.). Philadelphia: F.A. Davis

Torack, R.M. (1975): Congophilic angiopathy complicated by surgery and massive hemorrhage. Am. J. Pathol. 81, 349–366

Ulrich, G., Taghavy, A., Schmidt, H. (1973): Zur Nosologie und Ätiologie der kongophilen Angiopathie. Z. Neurol. 206, 39–59

Virchow, R. (1860): Cellular Pathology. London: J. Churchill

Weisenberg, R.C., Timasheff, S.M. (1970): Aggregation of microtubule subunit protein. Effects of divalent cations colchicine and vinblastine. Biochemistry 9, 4110–4116

Weiss, P. (1961): The concept of perpetual neuronal growth and proximo-distal substance convection In: Regional Neurochemistry. Kety, S.S., Elkes, J. (eds.). New York: Pergamon Press, pp. 220–242

Wilkins, R.H., Brody, I.A. (1969): Alzheimer's disease (Translation of; Über eine eigenartige Erkrankung der Hirnrinde. Centr. Nervenh. Psychiat. 30, 177–179, 1907). Arch. Neurol. 21, 109–110

Wilks, S. (1864): Clinical notes on atrophy of the brain. J. Ment. Sci. 10, 381–392

Wisniewski, H., Shelanski, M.L., Terry, R.D. (1964): Effects of mitotic spindle inhibitors on neuro-tubules and neurofilaments in anterior horn cells. J. Cell. Biol. 39, 224–229

Wisniewski, H., Narkiewicz, O., Wisnieska, K. (1967): Topography and dynamics of neurofibrillar degeneration in aluminum encephalopathy. Acta Neuropathol. 9, 127–133

Wisniewski, H., Terry, R.D. (1968): An experimental approach to the morphogenesis of neurofib-rillary degeneration and the argyrophilic plaque. In: Alzheimer's Disease and Related Conditions. Wolstenholme, G.E.W., O'Connor, M. (eds.). London: Churchill, pp. 223–241

Wisniewski, H.M., Johnson, A.B., Raine, C.S., Kay, W.J., Terry, R.D. (1970): Senile plaques and cerebral amyloidosis in aged dogs. Lab. Invest. 23, 287–296

Wisniewski, H., Terry, R.D., Hirano, A. (1970a): Neurofibrillary pathology. J. Neuropathol. Exp. Neurol. 29, 163–176

Wisniewski, H.M., Terry, R.D. (1973): Reexamination of the pathogenesis of the senile plaque. In Y Progress in Neuropathology. Zimmerman, H.M. (ed.). New York: Grune & Stratton, Vol. 2, pp. 1–26

Wisniewski, H.M., Ghetti, B., Terry, R.D. (1973): Neuritic (senile) plaques and filamentous changes in aged Rhesus monkeys. J. Neuropathol. Exp. Neurol. 32, 566–584

Wisniewski, H.M., Bruce, M.E., Fraser, H. (1975): Infectious etiology of neuritic (senile) plaques in mice. Science 190, 1108–1110

Wisniewski, H.M. (1975): Personal communication

Wisniewski, H.M., Narang, H.K., Terry, R.D. (1976): Neurofibrillary tangles of paried helical fila-ments. J. Neurol. Sci. 27, 173–181

Worster-Drought, C., Greenfield, J.G., McMenemey, W.H. (1940): A form of familial presenile dementia with spastic paralysis. Brain 63, 237–253

Worster-Drought, C., Greenfield, J.G., McMenemey, W.H. (1944): A form of familial presenile dementia with spastic paralysis. Brain 67, 38–43

7. Arteriosclerotic Dementia

Data obtained from records of acute and chronic hospitals and nursing homes often indicates a diagnosis of generalized cerebral arteriosclerosis which is merely a substitute for the proper diagnosis of senile or pre-senile dementia.

This diagnostic dilemma is compounded by the fact that advanced arteriosclerosis commonly in the same age groups as senile or even presenile dementia.

As a result, a pathogenetic hypothesis of "arteriosclerotic dementia" has been created that is highly questionable. It is certainly difficult, if not impossible, to support with clinical or laboratory data. There is no pathologic evidence to support the contention that occlusive cerebrovascular disease is a cause of neuronal degeneration leading to decline in intellect capacity only. (Fields, 1972.)

Although Fields was verbalizing sentiments shared by other investigators, this pronouncement created a shock of disbelief within the medical community. After all, arteriosclerosis has been the age-related disease that traditionally has been considered to be the best explanation of senile or presenile dementia other than premature aging. In other tissues, especially the kidney, the reduction of blood supply afforded by arteriosclerosis was considered to cause diffuse parenchymal damage leading to atrophy. Brain atrophy had been the most consistent manifestation of senile psychosis since Wilks in 1868, so it was quite natural to believe that cerebral arteriosclerosis was responsible for brain atrophy. This concept was formalized by Alzheimer (1899, 1902) and appeared as such in Kraepelin's seventh edition of *Psychiatrie* in 1904:

This psychosis appears about the sixtieth year; yet some cases develop before fifty, but in the latter instance there is usually present a strong hereditary tendency to vascular disease. When the disease occurs later in life, the arteriosclerosis may be associated with the characteristic senile changes of the nervous tissue which are dependent upon the vascular change. Alzheimer speaks of these cases as "Senile Decay". This form of disease attacks especially the cortical vessels that pass in from the pia, leading to the formation of deep wedge-shaped foci with destruction of the nerve tissue and an increase of glia.

An obsession with plaques and tangles resulted after the designation of Alzheimer's disease (AD) and interest in a vascular etiology declined proportionately. Alzheimer, the proponent of arteriosclerosis, became the champion of the new pathology. Even in 1934 when the nonspecificity of plaques and tangles was being recognized, Wertham and Wertham wrote disparagingly of arteriosclerosis as a cause of dementia:

"Cerebral arteriosclerosis" is not a clear-cut entity, either clinically or histopathologically. Contradictions, or seeming contradictions, exist everywhere. Some cases have hypertension; some, hypotension; still others, normal blood pressure. In some cases, the brain substance shows many "vascular lesions", i.e., lesions of a sort that can be produced only on a vascular basis — and yet the vessels are free from any demonstrable changes, and hypertension was not present while the patient was alive.

Rothschild seems to be very explicit in his denunciation of a vascular etiology of dementia when he discusses this relationship in 1942:

Structural damage to the brain is a constant feature and in some instances wholly accounts for the mental disorder. But in many instances the neuropathologic changes alone cannot satisfactorily explain the presence of a psychosis.

The concept of arteriosclerotic dementia has survived despite the critics from Alzheimer to Fields. The basis of such durability consists of two old and well-recognized facts. The first is the clinical nature of a vascular episode. Most frequently without warning, there is a functional deficit that subsequently improves but usually does not return to normal. The histories of demented patients are replete with a series of episodes of confusion and disorientation, after which the patient was never the same. The second is the pathologic evaluation of the cortex in arteriosclerosis by Alzheimer in 1902. In elderly psychotics he noted focal neuronal devastation (*Verödungen*) identical to the uninfarcted cortex in patients with multiple strokes. Macrovascular disease caused strokes; microvascular disease produced dementia. The only addition to this concept is the involvement of small arteries. Therefore three forms of cerebral arteriosclerosis have been considered important for dementia: (1) Large infarcts with clinically evident disability, (2) small infarcts that are clinically inconspicuous or silent, and (3) focal destruction of nerve cells without evidence of infarction.

Dementia Following Multiple Strokes

The most challenging aspect of stroke pathology is that it involves a focal structive lesion that facilitates clinicopathologic correlation. Therefore the symptoms of dementia should be correlated easily with distinct parts of the brain. Actually there are several distinctive aspects of arteriosclerotic psychosis. The most basic pattern was described by C. Miller Fischer (1968):

> In brief cerebrovascular dementia is a matter of strokes large and small. In most instances it will be evident from the tempo of events, combined with the occurrence of paralysis, sensory loss or visual field defect that a stroke has occurred. In many cases it is mental change not sensorimotor loss that prevents the patient from being restored to his place in the community of family.

The clinical criteria were defined more precisely by Roth (1955):

> Patients classified in this group (arteriosclerosis psychosis) were those (1) in whom dementia was associated with focal signs and symptoms indicative of cerebrovascular disease or (2) in whom a remittent or markedly fluctuating course at some stage of the dementing process was combined with any one of the following features; emotional incontinence, the preservation of insight or epileptiform seizures.

Hachinski (1974) adds an important consideration:

> Besides dementia, there are focal neurological signs and symptoms, a stepwise deterioration and often hypertension. The latter is stressed as a treatable aspect of the problem.

An important distinction is that the symptomatology of AD is more or less patterned, but in arteriosclerosis, infarcts can occur anywhere and the clinical correlates are equally randomized. Roth (1969) speaks about this diversity:

> No part of the brain is exempt from damage, however, and a variety of neurological syndromes may accompany the dementia. As well as hemiplegia, hemianopsia and aphasia already mentioned, apraxia, agnosia, epilepsy, pseudobulbar palsy and Parkinsonism may develop.

The most characteristic clinical aspect of arteriosclerotic dementia appears to be the stepwise deterioration accompanied by focal neurologic deficits. The dementia itself is largely indistinguishable from AD, but in this case, pathologic examination of the brain should be able to answer an important question. Is the dementia explained merely by greater destruction of brain; or is there a specific localization of brain destruction?

The pathologic correlation of strokes with dementing syndromes has been surprisingly sparse despite its early recognition and common occurrence. To be sure there are numerous descriptions of major vascular changes and a variety of cerebral softenings. Rothschild (1942) was the first to consider seriously the correlation between brain damage and dementia. The conclusions of this study are quite clear:

> In only a few cases were the cerebral changes so widespread that one might be inclined to stress the quantitative factor; in many instances the alterations were not extensive. There was no consistent correlation between the severity of the mental changes and the extent of the anatomic involvement.
> Thus, a scrutiny of the data without preconceived ideas indicates that even the impersonal aspects of the psychosis cannot be adequately explained by anatomic considerations alone.

After Rothschild we must wait for Corsellis (1962) who offered a distinction from senile dementia based on softening, plaques, and tangles. However this was chiefly a qualitative exercise and there was no attempt to explain the dementia by the size or distribution of the softening. Tomlinson (1970) has attempted to do both by an estimation of volume of brain softening and by an accurate localization of the infarcts. This important study reveals that only 9 of 50 senile dements were considered to represent "pure" arteriosclerotic dementia as characterized by the presence of brain softening and the absence of plaques and tangles.

The volume of brain damage varied between 60 and 412 ml. This tremendous variation of brain destruction was accompanied clinically by comparable levels of dementia. This seems to mean that the location of the infarcts in cases having smaller volumes is more critical than in brains with massive destruction:

> The emphasis on multiple basal ganglia and thalamic lesions in the descriptions of Rothschild (1942) and Coiffu (1958) appears unjustified; multiple lesions in these areas are not uncommon in non-demented patients but have not been the only, or even the predominant lesions in any case of arteriosclerotic dementia in this group. Massive ischaemic lesions, particularly involving brain supplied by middle or posterior cerebral arteries, were particularly significant. In the cases with more limited but still grossly visible lesions, occipito-temporal and hippocampal damage was often present, and in several, considerable lesions of the corpus callosum. (Tomlinson et al., 1970.)

Three cases had a volume of brain damage less than 101 ml (60, 71, 82) and in each of these there occurred prominent destruction of the corpus callosum and other areas of white matter. The occipitotemporal location was also mentioned by Rothschild (1942).

There appears to be little doubt that arteriosclerosis can cause dementia by a succession of brain-destructive episodes. These patients are characterized by a periodic occurrence of focal neurologic syndromes involving sensorimotor deficit and mental impairment. The dementia itself has no absolute distinction from AD. The pathologic correlate of this syndrome is a minimal volume of brain destruction of 60 ml with particular involvement of corpus callosum and terporooccipital lobes. Lesser degrees of softening are associated with dementia only when they occur concomitantly with plaques and tangles.

Little Strokes

Episodic confusion and disorientation in the elderly is almost always considered to be either a transient cerebral ischemia or a "little stroke". Actually little strokes are reputed to cause not only dementia but also a variety of disorders in the senium ranging from moral degeneration to tremor of the mandible. The concept of small or silent infarction is very real, being based upon the frequent occurrence of focal encephalomalacia at necropsy with no correlative clinical history of a stroke. In 1946 Alvarez pointed out that one should not expect the usual stroke symptomatology from such a small lesion. He considered instead that sudden, temporary, and repetitive clinical symptoms such as recurrent attacks of dizziness and fainting were the result of these tiny infarcts. That sounded quite reasonable.

The problem with little strokes was an overemphasis on their suddenness. When the restrictive criteria of transient and recurrent are ignored, any sudden change of life style in the elderly can be explained in this way:

> Often the thromboses occur during sleep. Diagnosis is fairly easy when the patient suddenly changes in character and ability. Some never work again. Many have an unexplained nervous break-down. Some become somewhat psychopathic and a difficult problem in the home. Some deteriorate morally. Occasionally one will go into a state of agitated depression. Many lose their grooming and go about with dirty clothing. Some fall unconscious. Some are overly emotional. Acute episodes are often thought to be attacks of "acute indigestion". (Alvarez, 1946.)

The pathologic equivalent to the small stroke is the lacunar infarct, which was described most thoroughly by Fisher (1969). The focal destruction is believed to be caused by segmental (small) arterial disorganization associated with hypertension. Most of these were found in silent areas of the brain and not associated with distinct clinical symptoms. However, when they occur in critical areas (e.g., in the brain stem, internal capsule) they have been linked quite clearly with clinical motor or sensory dysfunction. The real issue is whether small strokes can destroy 60 ml of tissue, which Tomlinson states is necessary for a causal relationship to elderly dementia. Fischer states, "There is no doubt that as the number of lucunes increases producing the lacunar state (or état lacunaire), mental deterioration does occur." All of the correlative problems that were present in relation to large strokes are relevant to small strokes. No one has ever demonstrated in a study analogous to that of Tomllinson et al. (1970) that a critical mass of tissue can be destroyed in this way to produce a dementing syndrome. Miller's statement is ambiguous at best. He means that there are cases of mental deterioration in which a large number of lacunes are present at necropsy.

There is no reason to question the entity of small cerebral infarcts, particularly occurring in hypertension. The chief problem appears to be an indiscriminate clinical overuse of little strokes as an explanation of sudden change in elderly behavior. The magnitude of this problem can be derived from pathologic studies of organic dementia (Tomlinson et al., 1970; Todorov et al., 1975; Corsellis, 1962). All agree that arteriosclerotic dementia is overdiagnosed and Corsellis estimates a 25% error. In a recent study of the anatomic correlate of transient ischemic attacks van der Drift and Kok (1972) found infarcts in 75% of their cases. It would appear that vascular disease is misdiagnosed in one out of four patients. The important aspect of this problem is that these patients probably represent AD and that the episodic confusion and disorientation should be a part of this clinical syndrome.

Diffuse Cerebral Ischemia

An ability to reduce brain function by a decrease in blood supply is a very old idea and actually carotid ligation was recommended as treatment for epilepsy by Burrows in 1848:

> The remarkable effects on the functions of the brain produced by ligature of the carotids or by other methods of obstructing the circulation through those vessels, have induced different persons to resort to such proceedings in the treatment of some cerebral disorders, such as epilepsy, which are almost incurable by other means.

Diffuse cerebral ischemia has been proposed as a result of macro- and microvascular disease. Carotid occlusive disease has been considered to be the chief large-vessel change that would cause diffuse cerebral ischemia and cortical atrophy. The microvascular correlate of ischemia is arteriolosclerosis as defined by Alzheimer. An essential feature of this ischemia regardless of cause is that it results in neuron degeneration but does not cause infarcts (complete destruction of tissue). Neurons are most susceptible to reduced blood flow because these cells have a higher metabolic rate and energy requirement than the other brain cells. A patchy perivascular nerve cell depletion was demonstrated by Alzheimer and is a fairly common finding in elderly brains. The precedent for selective neuron destruction are the lesions that occur in cardiac arrest, hypoglycemia, or anoxia in which neurons die but the glial cells and blood vessels remain.

Ischemia Due to Macrovascular Disease

Carotid Artery Occlusion

An etiologic relationship between progressive dementia and carotid occlusion was originated by Fisher (1951). In this report only one of three presented cases had a pathologic study that revealed numerous plaques and tangles in addition to bilateral occlusion. This association has become recognized as a fortuitous occurrence between two conditions that occur in the same age group because dementia in carotid occlusion has never been found without infarcts or in the absence of plaques and tangles. Endarterectomy has not proved beneficial in dementia therapy (Paulson et al., 1966), despite the improved blood flow that occurs after this procedure (Engell et al., 1972). By 1968, Fisher himself remarks, "This type of gradual loss of memory is not related to arteriosclerosis of the large and small cerebral arteries." This is exactly what Fields said 4 years later.

Vertebrobasilar Insufficiency

Unlike carotid disease, a dementing syndrome has consistently been included as a major complication of large vascular disease in the posterior circulation. Transient global amnesia was described by Fisher and Adams in 1964 and linked with vascular disease of the posterior circulation by Steinmetz and Vroom (1972). An evolution to permanent memory deficit and progressive dementia was postulated by Mathew and Meyer (1974). In these cases vertebrobasilar insufficiency has been established clinically on the basis of abnormalities seen by angiography and by regional reduction of cerebral blood flow. The actual development of infarcts seems to be less common and in these cases softening in the distribution of the posterior cerebral artery has been noted (Steinmetz and Vroom, 1972).

Another aspect of abnormal posterior circulation is the syndrome of "thalamic dementia", which has been related to disease of the rostral basilar artery (Segarra, 1970). This dementia has been characterized as a Korsakoff-like picture of memory deficit, an apathetic, indifferent lethargig state, which can terminate as akinetic mutism. In cases of akinetic mutism infarction of the medial dorsal nuclei of the thalamus can be found due to arteriosclerosis of the basilar artery and the posterior thalamosubthalamic paramedian artery.

Ischemia Due to Microvascular Disease

Alzheimer conceived arteriolosclerosis in the brain to be analogous to that of the kidney. In the kidney arteriolar thickening and renal atrophy are well recognized complications of arterial hypertension and a cerebral counterpart seems quite reasonable. The popularity of this concept suffered most by the revelation of plaques and tangles in progressive dementia. After all, Alzheimer himself had made the most visible conversion because he could not establish a relationship between thickened arterioles and the newly discovered plaques and tangles. Perhaps an even more serious defect in this concept is that arteriosclerosis has been reputed to be a frequent occurrence in aging unrelated to dementia. In this way arteriolosclerosis gradually assumed more significance for aging than for dementia but these changes may not be as widespread as generally believed, since McKeown (1975) found only 20% of her 90-year-olds to have such change. The final difficulty derives from the recognition that such arterioles become thickened secondary to atrophy of various cause. Despite all these contradictions, diffuse ischemia due to arteriolosclerosis as a cause of dementia had remained a viable concept until the studies of regional cerebral blood flow.

Cerebral Blood Flow Study of Dementia

The modern era of cerebral hemodynamics began when Kety and Schmidt (1948) developed the nitrous oxide method for quantitation of cerebral blood flow in man. The efficiency and accuracy of this system stimulated many studies on the effect of various stimuli, local and circulating, on cerebral blood flow. This work led to our current concept of autoregulation in which blood flow is adjusted to meet local metabolic and functional demands independent of the general circulation (Lassen, 1959; Sokoloff, 1959). Autoregulation is a function of the microcirculation; its effect is to minimize minor general changes in the macrovascular system such as hypertension and hypotension. This knowledge obviously was of great importance for any study of vascular disease. Suddenly a demonstration of vascular occlusion was not a sufficient correlate of ischemia, for it seemed possible that autoregulation could blunt its most deleterious effects.

Arteriosclerosis was the most logical objective for this type of study because its major effect is to reduce blood flow. The findings of Fazekas et al. (1953) were of momentous import:

The changes observed in cerebral blood flow, oxygen delivery, and cerebral vascular resistance were similar to but less marked than those previously noted for younger subjects with no evident cerebral vascular disease. Behavior of cerebral functions toward these several agents was essentially identical in both normotensive and hypertensive subjects. These findings indicate that even in the presence of cerebral arterisclerosis with or without hypertension the cerebral vasculature is capable of at least partial relaxation and conversely is sufficiently elastic to undergo a further increase of tonus in response to appropriate stimuli.

This study showed that autoregulation was still possible despite the vascular disease, so the abnormality must be limited to the larger arterial structures. In this way reactivity became an important factor in the evaluation of vascular disease. Using criteria of blood flow, oxygen consumption, and reactivity, a whole new classification of vascular disease was not only possible but necessary.

The study of organic dementia became urgent, since the vascular hypothesis of dementia was being revived following the collapse of morphology. The earliest study of psychoses in the elderly revealed concomitant reduction of blood flow and oxygen consumption (Freyhan et al., 1951):

Our data as a whole strongly suggest that the senile psychoses are associated with and probably the result of a significant reduction in cerebral oxygen utilization on the basis of an increased cerebrovascular resistance and its resultant significant reduction in blood flow through the brain. There is also no essential difference in this respect between the two clinical classifications of "psychosis with cerebral arterisclerosis" and "senile psychosis".

These conclusions indicated that Alzheimer was right about arteriolosclerosis and wrong about plaques and tangles.

The relationship of blood flow studies to aging and dementia was explored more thoroughly by Lassen et al. (1960), who not only confirmed the reduction of blood flow but also proposed that the decrease of oxygen consumption was an indicator of the degree of dementia. Sokoloff (1966) formalized the new concept of vascular dementia:

Decreases in cerebral blood flow and oxygen consumption are not the consequences of aging *per se* but rather of arteriosclerosis which causes first a relative circulatory insufficiency and hypoxia and then ultimately, after a protracted period of the latter, cerebral tissue damage and a reduction in cerebral metabolic rate.

About the only dissension with this viewpoint was that of O'Brien and Mallett (1970), who noted a reduction of blood flow in early secondary dementia (vascular disease) but not in early primary dementia (AD). In addition, Bower et al. (1970) could find no correlation between blood flow and the degree of dementia.

Probably the major problem with these studies is that they evaluated hemodynamics of the whole brain whereas in both AD and vascular disease regional alterations occur. This situation was corrected by the development of a practical method to study regional blood flow using a radioactive label, xenon 133, and multipe scintillation detectors arranged along various aspects of the cerebral hemisphere (Hoedt-Rasmussen et al. (1966). Regional reduction of blood flow in frontal and temporal areas was recognized immediately in AD and was correlated with normal reactivity of these blood vessels by Simard et al. (1971), who concluded:

This finding of normal vasomotor function in an unselected group of demented patients strongly supports the concept that dementia is not caused by long standing diminished blood flow due to cerebral atherosclerosis.

This means that blood supply is in equilibrium with the nutritive demand of the brain and that the diminished cerebral metabolism incident to atrophy evokes the reduction of blood flow. This concept was supported by the extensive survey of Gustafson and Risberg (1974) but they found the largest reduction of regional flow in the posterior temporal-occipital-parietal area. A distinction of multi-infarct dementia from AD was recently endorsed by Hachinski et al. (1975):

> The blood flow is adequate for metabolic needs of the brain in patients with primary degenerative dementia but inadequate for those with multi infarct dementia. There was no correlation between the degree of dementia and CBF (cerebral blood flow) in the primary degenerative group but an inverse relationship existed in the multi infarct group.

It seems appropriate to conclude that arteriosclerosis does not cause AD.

Summary

The participation of vascular disease in elderly dementia has been clarified significantly. Dementia can occur as a result of multiple infarction and cumulative brain destruction. The necessary volume (60 ml) and the location (corpus callosum, temporal and occipital lobe) seem to have been adequately defined. The potential of small strokes to produce this amount of brain destruction has never been demonstrated, so the theory that little strokes can produce dementia remains unproven. Diffuse cerebral ischemia causing dementia does not seem possible as a result of disease of the carotid circulation but it is a component of the clinical syndrome accompanying vertebro-basilar insufficiency. This seems to confirm Tomlinson's opinion that infarcts in the posterior circulation were more important than those of the anterior (carotid) circulation. The only exception would be the corpus callosum. The regional blood flow studies seem to have proven that AD does not have a vascular origin. In agreement with Fields, vascular disease appears to be overdiagnosed in dementia and generally such a diagnosis should not be made in the absence of clinically evident stroke.

References

Alzheimer, A. (1899): Beitrag zur pathologischen Anatomie der Seelenstörungen des Greisenalters. Neurol. Centralbl. 18, 95–96

Alzheimer, A. (1902): Die Seelenstörungen auf arterisklerotischer Grundlage. Allg. Z. Psychiatr. 59, 695

Alvarez, W.C. (1946): Cerebral arterisclerosis with small commonly unrecognized apoplexies. Geriatrics 1, 189–216

Bower, H.M, Andrews, J.T., Pope, R.A. (1970): Dementia and cerebral blood flow. Med. J. Aust. 1, 207–211

Burrows, G. (1848): Disorders of the Cerebral Circulation and on the Connection Between Affections of the Brain and Diseases of the Heart. Philadelphia: Lea and Blanchard

Corsellis, J.A.N. (1962): Mental Illness and the Aging Brain. Maudsley Monograph No. 9. London: Oxford Univ. Press

Engell, H.C., Boysen, G., Ladegaard-Petersen, H.J., Henriksen, H. (1972): Cerebral blood flow before and after carotid endarterectomy. Vasc. Surg. 6, 14–19

Evans, J.H. (1966): Transient loss of memory, an organic mental syndrome. Brain 89, 539–548

Fazekas, J.F., Bessman, A.N., Cotsonas, N.J., Alman, R.W. (1953): Cerebral hemodynamics in cerebral arteriosclerosis. J. Gerontol. 8, 137–145

Fields, W.S. (1974): Cerebral arteriosclerosis – a "non-cause" of dementia. In: Cerebrovascular Disease. 6th Int. Conf. 1972. Meyer, J.S., Lechner, H., Reivich, M., Eichhorn, O. (eds.). St. Louis: C.V. Mosby

Fisher, M. (1951): Senile dementia – a new explanation of its causation. Can. Med. Assoc. J. 65, 1–7

Fisher, C.M., Adams, R.D. (1964): Transient global amnesia. Acta Neurol. Scand. 40, (Suppl. 9), 7–82

Fisher, C.M. (1968): Dementia in cerebral vascular disease. In: Cerebral Vascular Diseases – 6th Conference. Siekert, R.G., Whisnant, J.P. (eds.). New York: Grune and Stratton

Fisher, C.M. (1969): The arterial lesions underlying lacunes. Acta Neuropathol. 12, 1–15

Freyhan, F.A., Woodford, R.B., Kety, S.S. (1951): Cerebral blood flow and metabolism in psychoses of senility. J. Nerv. Ment. Dis. 113, 449–456

Gustafson, L., Risberg, J. (1974): Regional cerebral blood flow related to psychoatric symptoms in dementia with onset in the presenile period. Acta Psychiat. Scand. 50, 516–538

Hachinski, V.C., Larssen, N.A., Marshall, J. (1974): Multi-infarct dementia. Lancet 2, 207–210

Hachinski, V.C., Iliff, L.D., Zilka, E., DuBoulay, G.H., McAllister, V.L., Marshall, J., Russell, R.W.R., Simon, L. (1975): Cerebral blood flow in dementia. Arch. Neurol. 32, 632–637

Holdt-Rasmussen, K., Sveinsdottir, E., Lassen, N.A. (1966): Regional cerebral blood flow in man determined by intra-arterial injection of radioactive inert gas. Circ. Res. 28, 237–247

Kraepelin, E. (1904): Lehrbuch der Psychiatrie. Translated by Diefendorf, A.R. New York: MacMillan, 1912

Lassen, N.A. (1959): Cerebral blood flow and oxygen consumption in man. Physiol. Rev. 39, 183–238

Lassen, N.A., Feinberg, I., Lane, M.H. (1960): Bilateral studies of cerebral oxygen uptake in young and aged normal subjects and in patients with organic dementia. J. Clin. Invest. 39, 491–500

MacKeown, E.F. (1975): De Senectute. J. R. Coll. Physicians Lond. 10, 79–99

Mathew, N.T., Meyer, J.S. (1974): Pathogenesis and natural history of transient global amnesia. Stroke 5, 303–311

O'Brien, M.D., Mallett, B.L. (1970): Cerebral cortex perfusion rates in dementia. J. Neurol. Neurosurg. Psychiatry 33, 497–500

Paulson, G.W., Kapp, J., Cook, W. (1966): Dementia associated with bilateral carotid artery disease. Geriatrics 21, 159–166

Roth, M. (1955): The natural history of mental disorder in old age. J. Ment. Sci. 101, 281–301

Roth, M., Myers, D.H. (1969): The diagnosis of dementia. Br. J. Hosp. Pract. 2, 705–717

Rothschild, D. (1942): Neuropathologic changes in arteriosclerotic psychoses and their psychiatric significance. Arch. Neurol. Psychiatry 48, 417–436

Segarra, J.M. (1970): Cerebral vascular diseaase and behavior. 1. The syndrome of the mesencephalic artery (Basilar artery bifurcation). Arch. Neurol. 22, 408–418

Simard, D., Odesen, J., Paulson, O.B., Lassen, N.A., Skinhoj, E. (1971): Regional cerebral blood flow and its regulation in dementia. Brain 94, 273–288

Sokoloff, L. (1959): The action of drugs on the cerebral circulation. Pharmacol. Rev. 11, 1–85

Sokoloff, L. (1966): Cerebral circulatory and metabolic changes associated with aging. Assoc. Res. Nerv. Ment. Dis. 61, 237–265

Steinmetz, E.F., Vroom, F.Q. (1972): Transient global amnesia. Neurology 22, 1193–1200

Todorov, A.B., Go, R.C.P., Constantinidis, J., Elston, R.C. (1975): Specificity of the clinical diagnosis of dementia. J. Neurol. Sci. 26, 81–96

Tomlinson, B.E., Blessed, G., Roth, M. (1970): Observations on the brains of demented old people. J. Neurol. Sci. 11, 205–242

Van der Drift, J.H.A., Kok, N.K.D. (1974): Clinical-pathological correlations in transient ischemic cerebral attacks. In: Cerebral Vascular Disease. 6th Int. Cong. Meyer, J.S., Lechner, H., Reivich, M., Eichhorn, O. (eds.). St. Louis, C.V. Mosby, pp. 187–192

Wertham, F., Wertham, F. (1934): The Brain as an Organ. New York: MacMillan

8. Critical Evaluation of the Concept of Mental Aging

The reality of finite existence is that every living species is programed for self-destruc-
tion. An endogenous lethal mechanism is demonstrated superbly by the death of the
Pacific salmon:

> A heavy rain or spate is generally required to drive the salmon upstream. At this time they are in
> prime condition, their bodies fat and oily, muscles taut, eyes keen.
> When they finally reach their destination the salmon prepare for the supreme ordeal of their lives.
> Every phase of their adventurous existence has led to this climax.
> After spawning both males and females live but a few days − none survives. Their spent, discolored,
> and rotting carcasses line the river or lake banks and are gnawed by wild animals and birds, drift
> downstream, or disintegrate where they perished, providing nutrients for the aquatic life the hatched-
> out fish will need to sustain their existence. (Netboy, 1974.)

Aging can be conceived as the sum of all inherent cellular events that combine to
result in the termination of life. Just as each species can be distinguished by a unique
pattern of aging, so each tissue has a characteristic relationship with time. The chronol-
ogy of brain life has been expressed in terms of intellectual function:

> The capacity to form comparisons and reason by analogy increases rapidly during childhood,
> appears to reach its maximum somewhere about the age of 14, after which it remains relatively con-
> stant until from about the age of 25 onwards it slowly declines. If the decline continues at a similar
> rate after the age of 60, it would appear that, by the age of about 80, the average person's capacity
> to grasp fresh ideas and adopt new methods of working has ceased to be greater than a child of eight.
> This is important in view of the fact that before the age of 8 years the average child is incapable of
> forming abstract comparisons and reasoning by analogy at least as a systematic method of learning.
> (Foulds and Raven, 1948.)

However, the littoral scene is not strewn with elderly subjects 80 or more having the
mentality of 8 year olds. Indeed major characteristing of mental aging is its variability,
which has been stressed by many observers from the aged Cicero in 44 *B.C.* (Couch,
1959): "All wines don't turn sour when they get old and neither do all men or all per-
sonalities," to Heron and Chown in 1967:

> Chronological age appears to be a familiar and reliable landmark: but "aging" may bring physical,
> physiological or psychological changes or may bring hardly any alteration in its wake. Individuals
> vary enormously at any given age in respect of almost all human characteristics. In the case of the
> characteristics studied here, the variation among individuals increases as the age of people studied
> increases. Indeed, this has been a finding in most work on aging, and makes any generalizations
> about "the aged" rather unsound.

The cause of such unpredictability is that the aging process is not the sole determinant of time-oriented function or death. Man, like most species other than salmon, has
aging mechanism that results in a decay of function but in practice rarely if ever causes
death. The relationship between aging and death has been described ably by Warthin (1928):

All of these factors are inherent within the germ plasm of the race; the individual's duration of life dependent upon such intrinsic factors is the normal or biologic span of life, and its termination constitutes normal or biologic death. But this is not the only form of death that may come to the multicellular animal organism, nor is it the usual one. Unfavorable factors in the environment may check the career of the individual at any time in its course – pathologic extrinsic death – the most common fate of animal life; or there may be present inherent abnormalities in the germ plasm of any given line foreordaining its early or premature termination – pathologic intrinsic death (inherited). Very few, if any, human beings achieve a biologic span of life and a normal intrinsic death; the great majority succumb to a pathological extrinsic death, a smaller number to a pathologic intrinsic death.

This distinction was conrimed most recently by MacKeown in her study of nonagenarians (1975):

Yet in considering the actual causes of death in the aged they are not very different from those found in younger geriatric groups.

Apart from identifying causes of death, this study fully confirms the multiplicity of disease processes in old age, some unrelated to each other, others interrelated, some combining to cause death, others being merely incidental. These diseases are ofteh superimposed on a background of a more general process of deterioration related to the involutionary changes associated with aging and which, it is claimed, increase the vulnerability of the elderly patient to disease, covering the lethal threshold for disorders that would have been of less consequence in younger age groups. However, since age changes alone are poorly defined and variable in their time of onset – and indeed there is doubt as to what descent they are uncomplicated expressions of senescence – their influence on the evolution of disease is far from clear.

It is apparent that a major problem for any investigator of function in the elderly is the question of whether altered performance is due to age or to an age-related disease. This is especially true of the brain and it constitutes the reason for the continuous debate regarding arteriosclerosis and aging as the cause of dementia. The obvious prerequisite for such a judgment is a clear concept of mental aging.

An effect of time on the brain has been predicated on the fact that old people slow down and have small brains. Particularly within the past 10 years, this has stimualted a massive study of mental function, brain chemistry, and brain structure, which has been reviewed recently by Ordy and Brizzee (1975) and Maletta (1974). Our modern concept of brain aging derives from our current appreciation of performance of the elderly brain and of the physical changes in the organ following death.

The general hypothesis proclaims an age-related relentless loss of brain tissue beginning at age 25 (Appel and Appel, 1942) which is due primarily to death of nerve cells (Brody, 1955). No one has ever shown that this decline is not linear. Therefore, at some point, it must be correlated with reduced brain function. This is precisely what Foulds and Raven (1948) had in mind and the correction for variability does not alter the validity of the premise that mental decay occurs with time. The vital questions that require clarification include (1) the manifestation of this neuron loss in terms of altered brain function, (2) the biologic significance of the changes in the brain organ, and (3) the usefulness of these abnormalities as indicators of early or accelerated mental aging. The latter state is synonymous with dementia or Alzheimer's disease (AD).

Functional Aspects of the Elderly Brain

Mental Behavior in the Aged

Memory

I'm not a bit worried by the popular saying "Read tombstones and lose your memory". It is by reading those very stones that I refresh my memory of the dead. And really I have never heard of any old
man forgetting where he had buried his treasure; the old remember what is of real concern to them:
their days in court, their debts, and their debtors. (Cicero, 44 *B.C.*)

There is little doubt that defective memory is the most common complaint of senior
citizens. Defective memory has been shown to occur as early as the 5th decade (Hamilton, 1938) and after 65 at least 80% of the population appear to have some impairment
(Bot winnick and Storandt, 1974). There appears to be overwhelming evidence that the
memory problem associated with aging involves recent rather than remote memory.
These two facets of memory achieve distinction not only because of their selective
decline in aging but also because of their characteristic evolution during childhood
(Campbell and Spear, 1972). In the latter situation recent memory appears vigorous yet
human experiences prior to age 5 are largely unavailable for recall by the adult individual.
Moreover at any age, a selective, temporary defect of recent memory is common as a
result of physical or even emotional trauma, which will not affect remote memory
(Russell, 1959).

The neurobiology of memory has been the subject of much recent research and appears to involve at least three distinct mechanisms: (1) A recognition of new information that is initially presented to the CNS by any one of the specialized systems of sensory perception. (2) A registration of this data that is accomplished in such a way as to
be available for appropriate use at some future date. (3) The retrieval of the stored information, which occurs at the desire of the individual.

In the aged, the basis of recent memory loss has been difficult to establish because
there are multiple factors relating to memory. Recognition is complicated by decay of
various sensory function (Corso, 1975), by decreased attention span (Misky and Harmon, 1974) and by greater individual discrimination regarding meaningful information,
i.e., that which is worthy of storage (Botwinnick and Storandt, 1974). Furthermore
psychometric assay of memory has resulted in a belief that the storage mechanisms differ for long- and short-term memory but there is no explanation for the selective decline
of the latter. Retrieval appears to be intact; in fact, the avowal by many elderly that
they remember facets of remote memory better may be an indication of even more
efficient retrieval. So the problem of recent memory probably accrues from defective
reception or inadequate storage or both.

The recognition of a modulating effect upon these memory mechanisms by various
drugs has stimulated studies of learning and retention in laboratory animals (Gold and
McGaugh, 1975). A significant aspect of these studies is that they enhance the contention that the processes underlying short- and long-term memory are different (McGaugh
and Herz, 1972). Acquisition and retention of learned responses can be facilitated by
drugs affecting adrenergic mechanisms, cholinergic mechanisms, and the synthesis of
RNA (McGaugh, 1973). Other chemical and physiologic treatments have been shown
to have a deleterious effect on memory (Jarvik, 1972).

A most important aspect of memory loss is that, in most old people, it is not progressive and remains restricted to a recollection of recent information (Klonoff and Kennedy, 1974). Very few investigators have noted any predictive value for memory loss, unless it is associated with vascular disease (strokes) or with AD (Goldfarb, 1975). Botwinnick (1967) has noted that, in surviving males, memory declines less than in females after the age of 80. This may reflect a survival of the fittest, since the less adequate males have succumbed at an earlier age. Only Kral (1967) has proposed a predictive value for memory loss, which he characterizes as forgetfulness of recent events in addition to persons, places, or dates. It may be of interest that his finding of 50% mortality within 4 years was not related to dementia, but rather to a collapse of stress mechanisms. The proposed relationship between adrenergic mechanisms and memory would support this concept. As a final note, there is rather general agreement that the anatomic basis for senescent memory loss is the degeneration of the hippocampus represented by senile plaques and neurofibrillary tangles. However Tomlinson et al. (1968) found no such change in 11 of 28 nondemented persons aged 65–92 years of age.

Cognitive Function

The entire area of cognitive decline with aging has become very confused for a variety of reasons.

1. Many early studies showing such decay were not designed to compensate for increases of reaction time commonly found in the elderly (Baer, 1971).
2. Decrements of sensory function were frequently not admitted by such subjects and consequently they were not tested specifically, Some of these defects are related to receptor defects but others are considered to have a central origin (Corso, 1975).
3. Reevaluation of intelligence data using longitudinal as well as cross-sectional analysis has revealed a reversal of some cognitive defects that were noted in the cross-sectional surveys (Shaie, 1970). At least one such longitudinal survey has suggested that survival of high performers was responsible for this change (Riegel et al., 1967).
4. There has been a distinct correlation between cognitive decline and general body disorder such as hypertension and vascular disease (Wilkie and Eisdorfer, 1971).

At this time there appears to be no way in which meaningful conclusions can be derived from the existing data. Nonetheless cognitive decline does appear to be part of the aging process. This impasse has been well summarized by Sherkin (1974):

> The higher cognitive functions of problem solving and creativity decline with age, slowly in the healthy and more rapidly in those with poor health. Severe decrements reflect normal aging plus age related conditions such as impaired perceptual and memory abilities and reduced psychomotor speed. In the absence of such conditions, or when test scores are adjusted for them cognitive function remains functional into the eighties. Dissection of cognition into its component factors, and analysis of their changes with time, may lead to identification of the predominant determinants of cognitive defects in the normal aged and in the average aged.

Psychoses After 65

The initial onset of a reversible psychotic episode in old age has been regarded as another aspect of brain aging until the various psychotic disorders of aging were defined by Roth (1955). We have noted already (Chapt. 1) how the early organists and the later Freudians distinguished functional disease in the elderly from that of the young. Roth (1955) showed clearly that the outcome in functional psychoses and paraphrenia was distinct from that of arteriosclerotic and senile psychosis and that there was no different hereditary influence in functional disease before or after the age of 60. Kay et al. (1964) showed that age was a factor in the occurrence of organic psychosis but not in functional disease but the following comment left room for doubt:

Yet these features (of the elderly) — bereavement, reduction in contacts and physical disability — are not in themselves sufficient causes of psychiatric illness; their traumatic effects depend on a pre-existing disability.

A reasonable possibility is that the age-related loss of neurons is the basis of this predisposition. Age-related changes in parasympathetic and sympathetic networks have been appreciated by Nelson and Gelhorn (1958) and have been considered the basis for some of the different therapeutic effects seen in the elderly (Bender, 1970). This may be related to the decrease in aging of both dendritic spines (Sheibel et al., 1975) and of synapses (Cragg, 1975), which would be a logical accompaniment of neuronal cell loss. Perhaps the strongest argument for some organic factor in functional disease is the finding by Post (1962) of affective symptoms in 69% of patients with arteriosclerotic or senile psychosis, either at the time of initial examination or within the following 6 years.

Despite such evidence for an age factor, the behavior of patients with long-standing functional disorder belies its existence. Age-related changes would be expected to aggravate existing disease if they were of etiologic significance. Yet Muller (1971) has noted that 46 of 101 chronic schizophrenics "had become more reasonable, clearer, harder workers, who demonstrated better object relations and even showed insight into their former pathological state." This would appear to confirm the previous findings of Ciompi (1969), who noted improvement in both neurotic and depressive symptoms but some aging effect was suggested by their "replacement with different affective disorders and residual states." A reasonable conclusion is that there is no evident identification of an aging factor in the occurrence of functional mental disease in the elderly. The huge incidence (25%–35%) is believed to result from the physical, social, and economic stresses of this age (Bergmann, 1972).

Electroencephalography

Routine EEG

The EEG, in conjunction with psychological testing and blood flow study, form the triad of measures that have been used to characterize brain function in aging throughout the past 30 years. At the beginning of this period, definitive intellectual decline was considered to occur as early as 30 years of age (Sect. 3). If aging caused such a change in global function, it was most reasonable to believe that there would be an electrical correlate to aid in early diagnosis and a vascular defect to explain the cause of mental decay. In this way, these tests were used not only as indices of aging but also or parallel function, i.e., the EEG as a measure of intelligence.

The elderly EEG demonstrates several abnormalities, the chief of which are slowing and amplitude reduction of alpha waves. These changes of alpha activity have been described both in the temporal lobe (Mundy-Castle, 1951) and in the occipital lobe (Obrist, 1963). There is also a tendency to develop theta and delta activity, which can be diffuse but more commonly is focal and located in the temporal lobe (Kooi et al., 1964). In addition fast beta activity has been described with increasing incidence up to age 80 (Busse and Wang, 1965) but this has been debated (Mankovsky and Belonog, 1971).

The significance of these abnormalities has been controversial because of their inconsistency and because of their poor predictive value. No evidence of EEG abnormality can be noted in anywhere from 35% (Mengoli, 1952) to 80% (Obrist, 1963) of the elderly population. More important was the variability of repetitive testing. Sheridan et al. (1955) studied his subjects every 3 months for 2 years and reported:

> It is exceptional for serial recordings to remain unchanged. These changes consist of increase or decrease in the basic alpha rhythm; change in general integration, change in amount of slow activity, presence or absence of paroxysmal dysrhythmia, change in symmetry, variation in hyperventilation response; and change in location, quantity and quality of focal activity.

Nevertheless the abnormal EEG was considered to have predictive value until Obrist (1972) showed no decreased longevity or abnormal intellectual decline in these subjects after 12 years of study.

The whole relationship between the EEG and psychometrics has been debatable (Egglingson, 1966; Vogel and Broverman, 1966) but Busse and Obrist (1963) could find no difference in the test performance of elderly subjects with or without EEG changes. There was also no correlation between abnormal EEG and reduced hemispheral blood flow (Obrist et al., 1963). The advent of regional blood flow permitted a more sophisticated comparison of blood flow and focal EEG changes (Ingvar et al., 1965) particularly of the temporal lobe. No report of such correlation exists. At the present time, EEG abnormalities have no distinct relationship to brain aging. Perhaps the best evidence that these alterations have no malignant implication is the recent report of EEGs in centenarians (Hubbard et al., 1976) in which 8 out of 10 subjects had the same variety of changes described in younger elderly. There was no evidence of greater slowing than that occurring at age 80.

Visual Evoked Response (VER)

The measurement of visually evoked cortical responses may have greater significance for aging than the routine EEG. These potentials, which are generated by the occipital lobe, have been shown to undergo various changes between 1 month and 81 years (Dustman and Beck, 1969). Decreasing amplitude, increased latency of response and the presence of new components seem to characterize visual evoked response (VER) in the elderly (Dustman and Beck, 1969; Straumanis et al., 1965). A correlation between VER and intelligence has been reported (Shucard and Horn, 1972; Weinberg, 1969) with particular relevance to verbal intelligence (Weinberg, 1969). There has been report of concurrent assay of occipital blood flow and VER so any vascular relationship is indefinite at this time.

The changes related to aging differ from those that have been reported in AD (Visser et al., 1976) and Creutzfeldt-Jakob disease (Lee and Blair, 1973). Although VER were originally described in 1934 by Adrian and Matthews they have received little attention until their relationship to organic disease was reported. Therefore it appears prudent to suspend judgment on the specificity of these changes for aging and disease until they are corroborated by other investigators.

Cerebral Blood Flow

There have been three distinct aspects of cerebral blood flow assays relative to aging (1) global studies using the nitrous oxide method of Kety and Schmidt (1945), (2) regional blood flow studies using intra-arterial xenon (Hoedt-Rasmussen et al., 1966) and (3) longitudinal studies.

Very soon after the introduction of the nitrous oxide method a reduction of blood flow and oxygen consumption was noted in aged subjects (Fazekas et al., 1952). The significance of this finding was clarified quickly by the same group (Fazekas et al., 1953), who studied a group of 18 subjects between the ages of 90 and 102. In this study, the blood flow and metabolic rate of the nonagenarians was significantly lower than that occurring in individuals younger than 50 but not statistically different from a group of elderly people having a mean age of 69 years. This seemed to indicate that age-related changes did not correlate with the progression of atrophy and neuron loss.

The regional blood flow studies in normal young individuals revealed a lower fast component in the temporal lobes whereas the slow component was about equal throughout (Ingvar et al., 1965). There has been no report of a study designed solely to study aging effects but Ingvar and Schwartz (1974) report normal flow in 10 subjects aged 31–68 and Wilkinson et al. (1969) report normal flow in 10 subjects aged 18–64. Since the study of Ingvar and Schwartz is sensitive enough to reveal altered flow patterns in speech production it seems safe to assume that aging has no effect on regional blood flow in man.

Two longitudinal surveys of aging have included blood flow measurement with an attempt to correlate blood flow and intellectual ability. In the NIH study Dastur et al. (1963) found no difference between a group of healthy aged subjects (mean age 70.8 years) and a group of young controls (mean age 20.8 years) that could correlate with EEG changes and diminished performance in intellectual testing. However there was a significant decrease of blood flow in a group of men (mean age 72.4 years) who had asymptomatic cardiovascular disease. Accordingly they concluded that the vascular disease and not aging per se was the cause of this change. When this same group was evaluated in 1967 there was no significant relationship of mortality to any parameter of vascular dynamics other than mean arterial blood pressure (Libow et al., 1971). In the Duke longitudinal study "the only statistically significant correlation (WAIS), however, was that between blood flow and performance change in the group with high educational and socioeconomic status" (Wang et al., 1974). This correlation has dubious significance, since many personal and environmental factors in this group have a similar relationship. Therefore the results of all types of assay appear to be in agreement that there is no abnormality of cerebral blood flow that can be used as a criterion of aging or as an indicator of intellectual decline and premature death.

Immunologic Indices of Aging

The immunology theory of aging was formally proposed by Walford in 1969;

Aging is due to somatic cell variation, particularly of those factors which determine self-recognition patterns among cells. In higher animals the cells of the reticulo-endothelial system are especially involved. Aging in these species is brought about by the unleashing of self-destroying processes of the nature of auto immunity or transplantation disease. The initial cause of the somatic cell variation whatever it may be, is extrinsic to this pathogenetic mechanism although this variation may be further stimulated by auto-catalytic immune processes.

In effect Walford is saying that imperfect cells are being produced throughout the life of the organism but that only the perfect cells survive destruction by an alert immune antibody system, which recognizes and eliminates the defective cells. As this immune mechanism deteriorates with age, these imperfect cells are allowed to live, perhaps even proliferate, and eventually effect a decline in composite function plus a premature death. The application of this concept to the aging brain was hindered by two facts: (1) Neurons are postmitotic cells with limited potential for cell variation and (2) the brain is an immunologically privileged site due to the macromolecular vascular barrier. However, the more accurate definition of the magnitude of neuronal cell loss with aging emphasized a need to understand self-destructive cell processes better. Furthermore, the recognition of the immunoglobulin nature of amyloid, which is so common in aging brain, caused doubt regarding the effectiveness of the immunologic privilege in aging.

Since 1969, there has occurred a great sophistication of this concept and at present the sequence of events proposed by Walford is quite controversial. The extrinsic cause of somatic variation could just as easily result in somatic cell destruction without an antibody reaction. Furthermore antibody synthesis has been noted to be maintained even in the face of diminished cellular immune function. Recently Adler (1974) has presented a revised immunologic concept of aging in which diminished cellular immune function is correlated with recurrent viral infections:

> With repeated viral infections, starting possibly at conception, the individual acquires a "library" of viral genetic information. Concurrently, the cell-mediated immune system undergoes a decline in activity. Viral infected tissue that cannot be policed by lymphocytes is attached by anti-viral antibody or anti-tissue antibody and the phenomena of auto-antibody becomes manifest. Virus plus antibody results in immune complex disease, but not in a rejection of diseased tissue. The infections continue causing normal tissue disease.

The most consistent aspect of these studies is that there is a decreased level of activity of the immune system probably related to the number of immunocompetent cell units (Makinodan et al., 1971), which is associated with abnormal lymphocyte function (Weksler and Hutteroth, 1974). A recent study by Roberts-Thomson et al. (1974) has revealed that lymphocyte responses are quite reduced in some old people. Most impressive is their statistic of 80% mortality in this group within 2 years. On the other hand, antibody production may be increased (Walford, 1965), normal (Adler et al., 1971), or decreased (Haferkamp et al., 1966). Specific antibody may be antiviral or antitissue. Therefore the role of immunity in aging has numerous mechanisms, each with vast importance.

The relevance for brain aging remains more potential than real. Brain-specific antigens have been identified in short-term cultures (Bock et al., 1975). Brain-reactive antibodies were identified in the serum of aged mice (Threatt et al., 1971), which have been claimed to be specific for neuronal antigen (Nandy et al., 1975). The major effort to study serum immunoglobulins has been that of Buckley et al. (1974) in the Duke longitudinal study of aging. Surviving older subjects have demonstrated a gradual elevation of serum IgG and IfA, while decreased serum immunoglobulins were correlated with mortality.

In summary we have very limited knowledge of immunologic indices of brain aging. Neuronal cell loss could be due to an antigenic mechanism that is triggered by the early death of superfluous or noncompetent neurons. The amyloid in senile plaques could indicate an altered immune system in the aging brain. The concept that aging represents altered response to viral infection may have great significance for the occurrence of Creutzfeldt-Jakob disease.

Pathology of the Aged Brain

Brain Weight as a Determinant of Atrophy

The three inevitable consequences of human social existence are taxes, death, and brain atrophy. This statement is obviously false. Henry David Thoreau would be the first to repudiate the necessity of taxes and anyone can avoid brain atrophy by dying before the age of 25. But we have noted already how atrophy has been considered both the hallmark of aging and of dementia (Sect. 1). The similarity in the patterns of brain loss has been a major component of the concept that dementia is exaggerated aging. The atrophic process has been recognized to result in a decrease in brain wieght as early as 1880 by Bischoff. The early studies of age-related weight loss were reviewed by Pearl in 1905 and revealed a linear regression between the ages of 15 and 80. Appel and Appel (1942) found a similar linearity, which they extended to age 96. They also noted that by 96 slightly more than 10% of the brain had vanished. The unfortunate aspect of this study is that their brains were obtained from a mental hospital. More recently Burger (1954), Hoch-Ligeti (1963), and Peress et al. (1973) have observed a similar decrement with age so that there is no reason to doubt the validity of this finding.

An important aspect of all these studies is that the brain weight for any given age is a mean that has been derived from a varying number of brains. Therefore it is the "average brain weight" that diminishes with age. This has been interpreted to mean that all of us are programed to lose 10% of our brain by 90 and more if we are fortunate enough to survive. Yet this is not really true, since it is well recognized that female brains weight less but do not have the same degree of weight loss (Peress et al., 1973; Burger, 1954). This suggestion that weight loss is not the same in all brains is enhanced by the realization that the minimum brain weight (Table 8.1) in the series of Appel and Appel (1942) did not change between 25 and 96. The dubious nature of the brains used in their study has prompted a re-evaluation of Pearl's data. The variation of brain weight at the various age groups has been compiled from his statistics and is shown in Table 8.2. The minimum brain weight is strikingly uniform at all ages especially in males, and this is very comparable to the data of Appel and Appel (Table 8.1). There is a definite reduction in the maximum brain weight so the decreasing mean brain weight seems to accrue from weight loss involving the larger brains.

This concept of differential decline in brain mass is most important. It must mean that a brain with minimal weight at age 25 will be the same at 55 or 95. This indicates that the loss of nerve cells is not a random process common to all individuals. If the 1000-g brain can be conceived to represent the least amount compatible with our evolutionary state, it must also be considered to represent critical mass. By corollary, aging is not affecting this critical mass, it is affecting brain tissue in excess of this mass. Therefore it appears that aging is a process that primarily involves a destruction of superfluous

Table 8.1. Variation in brain weight with age (non-lesioned-brain cases) (Appel and Appel, 1942)

Age classes (years)	No. of cases	Range (grams)
12–24	19	870–1700
25–29	61	1050–1600
30–34	105	1060–1660
35–39	109	1050–1634
40–44	141	936–1750
45–49	151	1020–1729
50–54	182	1046–1720
55–59	164	990–1720
60–64	199	950–1690
65–69	257	1000–1700
70–74	303	972–1620
74–79	223	934–1550
80–84	126	971–1560
85–96	39	1050–1400

Table 8.2. Variation in brain weight of Hessians, Bavarians, and Swedes (Pearl, 1905)

Age class	Males		Females	
	No.	Range	No.	Range
25–29	143	1100–1749	94	1050–1599
30–34	167	1050–1699	89	900–1499
35–39	177	1050–1699	103	1050–1499
40–44	155	1000–1649	82	1000–1549
45–49	123	1000–1649	66	950–1449
50–54	163	1000–1749	76	800–1449
55–59	117	1100–1699	63	1050–1449
60–64	92	1000–1649	58	950–1399
65–69	67	1000–1599	43	900–1399
70–74	38	1100–1599	43	800–1399
75–79	25	1000–1499	16	950–1299

nerve cells and not critical or necessary nerve cells. This may be the most important thing we have ever learned about brain aging.

Programed destruction is also evident in the predilection of certain parts of the brain for atrophy. In this regard the frontal poles and the temporal lobes have consistently been regarded as the sites of most prominent shrinkage (Critchley, 1931). Moreover the grey matter, represented by the cortical ribbon, has been recognized to suffer most by this process. This implies that the neuron is primarily affected, since it is the unique cellular component of grey tissue. White matter atrophy has traditionally been viewed as a secondary event caused by a loss of myelinated axons that derive from the affected nerve cells. Enlargement of ventricles is believed to be a consequence of reduction in white matter volume.

Neuron Loss With Aging

The neuronal involvement in atrophy has been confirmed by qualitative descriptions of cell loss dating at least to Alzheimer, and more recently by quantitative counts of neurons in microscopic preparations. This latter procedure is not usually considered dignified utilization of cortical function, so man has devised a machine, the image analyzer, which has freed him of this onerous chore (Henderson et al., 1975). There is now good evidence to show that the temporal lobe is particularly vulnerable to neuron loss.

The quantification of cortical neurons in aging has been reported by Brody (1955), Colon (1972), and Shefer (1972). The most complete study is that of Brody, since Shefer counted only the third cortical layer, while Colon examined only one area of cortex. Colon states that 45% of the neurons die by age 80. Shefer has compared 5 subjects (19–28 years of age) with 10 elderly (mean age 77 years) and found a decrement of 22%–29% with the greatest decrease in the temporal lobe (subiculum). Brody evaluated neurons in 20 brains varying in age from newborn to 95 years. According to Brody, the most convincing neuronal depletion occurs in the superior temporal gyrus, where a progressive decline is noted between the ages of 16 and 95 resulting in a 55% loss. Similar rough estimates show that there is a 40% decrease in the precentral gyrus, a 20% loss in the occipital lobe, and no loss in the postcentral gyrus (Brody, 1955).

In addition to these studies of neocortex, quantitative assays have involved the inferior olive (Moatamed, 1966; Monagle and Brody, 1971), ventral cochlear nucleus (Konigsmark and Murphy, 1970), cerebellum (Ellis, 1919, 1920; Hall et al., 1975), and the spinal nerve roots (Gardner, 1940). No decrease in the cell population of the inferior olive could be noted between birth and age 85 (Monagle and Brody, 1971) or between birth and age 56 (Moatamed, 1966). Konigsmark could find no neuron loss in the ventral cochlear nucleus between 4 months and 90 years. The loss of Purkinje cells is unquestioned, but Ellis (1919) noted a 50% loss while Hall et al. (1975), using more sophisticated techniques, have reported only a 25% decrease. Ellis (1920) also noted a loss of neurons in the dentate nucleus despite the prominent accumulation of pigment. Gardner found a 20% reduction in the number of fibers in spinal roots between ages 34 and 85.

These studies certainly confirm the concept of neuronal destruction accompanying age and the idea that this is not a random process. Since this had been known previously, it would be desirable to have new information such as some indication of why some nerve cells die and others do not. There is some suggestion that phylogenetically new areas of the brain are less susceptible to cell loss than the older regions. This is best indicated by the disparity between precentral and postcentral gyrus, since only the rostral margin of the postcentral gyrus would be included in the mesopallium (Yakovlev, 1948). However, the superior temporal gyrus has an evolution similar to the postcentral gyrus and has the greatest cell loss. Moreover, the inferior olive is completely mesopallial and shows no decrement with age. Neuronal systems are also considered to have common metabolic pathways, which could serve as a basis or preferential decay. In this way precentral gyrus and anterior spinal root involvement would appear to be linked but there is no similar correlation between nerve fiber loss in posterior (sensory) spinal roots and the postcentral gyrus. Furthermore the disparity between Purkinje cell loss and depletion in the dentate nucleus plus the integrity of the inferior olive is inconsistent with such a viewpoint.

A vascular basis is suggested by the lower vascular supply of the temporal and occipital areas in comparison to that of the frontal and pararolandic fissure areas (Ingvar et al., 1965). Temporal and occipital lobe depletion could be explained on this basis but the difference between pre- and postcentral gyrus is inexplicable, since both have similar blood flow values. The lack of any demonstrable defect in regional blood flow in aging, particularly of the temporal lobe, would also contradict such a hypothesis.

A rational argument for the loss of superfluous neurons has been derived from the brain weight data; however, at present we have no means of identifying these cells. Sex and stature have been the two chief correlates of increased brain weight, so muscle mass seems to be one determinant of greater neuron number. Perhaps the decline of physical prowess with age is a factor in neuron depletion in the motor cortex. The next consideration is that "silent" areas like the frontal lobes would be largely affected. But the complexitiy of this problem is illustrated by the fact that the superior frontal gyrus has only 8% more cell loss than the very necessary precentral gyrus (Brody, 1970). Only one other aspect of this impass is known at this time: that brain weight does not correlate with intelligence.

Although we do not know why these cells die, the distinctiveness of the neuron loss in aging should be useful in establishing a similarity or difference between aging and dementia. There are three reports of comparative neuron counts in aging and dementia (Shefer, 1972; Ball, 1976; Terry, 1977) and unfortunately the results differ. Shefer (1972) counted only the third cortical layer, but found that the pattern of cortical cell loss in dementia differed from that of aging. Terry (1977) found that the cell loss is identical in aging and dementia. However Terry did not count the hippocampus, where both Shefer (1972) and Ball (1976) have noted a distinctive cell loss in dementia. At this point, the cell counts support the contention that senile dementia ia a disease of the limbic system that is distinct from aging of the neocortex.

Senile Plaques, Neurofibrillary Tangles, Granulovacuolar Degeneration

The progressive nature of neuronal loss in aging implies that at any age some of the surviving cells will also die by the same mechanism, particularly in areas of greatest cell loss. We have noted already how senile plaques (SP), neurofibrillary tangles (NF), and granulovacuolar degeneration (GVD) were associated with aging neurons (Sect. 1). Since none of these is specific for aging, an etiologic relationship can be established only if they occur predominantly in areas of greatest neuron loss. Quantitative assays are optimally designed to answer this question.

The best study of this type is by Tomlinson et al. (1968) who counted SP, NF, and GVD in the same cortical areas (precentral, postcentral, striate, superior temporal) that were studied by Brody (1955). In addition they added the hippocampus and hippocampal gyrus. Some of the results of this study are shown in Table 8.3, which has been formulated from information in the report (Tomlinson et al., 1968). The most surprising aspect of this work is that SP appear more prominently in the occipital lobe than in the temporal lobe. When greater numbers of plaques (more than eight) were found, all areas of cortex were involved, but in three cases, most SP occurred in the frontal lobe and in two cases they were predominantly occipital. Frontal involvement was also conspicuous when five or less plaques per field were noted but, with only scattered plaque involvement,

Table 8.3. Distribution of morphologic changes in nondemented elderly (compiled from Tomlinson et al., 1968)

	Frontal	Parietal	Occipital	Temporal	Hippocampal
SP $<$ 1/field		1	5		
SP $<$ 6/field	3	1	1	2	5
SP $>$ 8/field	3		2		
NF (all)	1	1	3	1	16
GV					10

SP, senile plaques; NF, neurofibrillary tangles; GV, granulovascular change.

the occipital lobe again was the most likely site. The occipital lobe was also the neocortical area most likely to have NF although the hippocampus was the predominant location of NF. GVD were only found in the hippocampus. Tomlinson et al. have not emphasized this point but it is obvious that the occurrence of these abnormalites does not correlated with the areas of greatest neuronal loss reported by Brody (1955). It is unfortunate that the hippocampus, a chief site of involvement, was not studied by Brody. The most extensive study of the hippocampus was reported by Ball (1976), who noted an aging effect only in the anterior half, whereas in dementia the posterior half was also altered. This new loss of neurons was not of the same degree of magnitude as the incidence of NF.

Lipofuscin

The accumulation of lipofuscin during the life of many animal cells has been recognized for over 100 years. The early investigators of senility and AD (Sect. 1, Table 1.1) all mention prominent neuronal aggregates of lipofuscin but they do not accord etiologic significance equal to that of SP or NF. However in 1959, Strehler et al. were searching for a marker of cellular aging and they believed that lipofuscin fulfilled their four criteria of aging, universality, time dependence, intrinsicality, and deleteriousness. Since that time much interest has focused on lipofuscin both as a marker and as a pathogenetic mechanism of cell aging and death.

The first three criteria of Strehler et al. (1959) probably are fulfilled by lipofuscin. Although there is a great disparity in individual neuronal content, it seems likely that every neuron makes some lipofuscin (Torack, 1976); at least no one has shown serial electron micrographs of a neuron without a single lipofuscin granule. There is no question about the increase of lipofuscin accumulation with age, but the early onset of neuronal pigment, which can be found even in aborted fetuses (Humphrey, 1944), may create skepticism regarding its validity as a marker of age. The aspect of intrinsicality is satisfied with a fairly general acceptance of the pigment granule as a type of autophagic lysosome. In this context it would be part of the neuronal degradative system that breaks down a variety of cellular debris. The end result is lipofuscin, which is not turned over rapidly and tends to accumulate with age.

The major objection to the lipofuscin hypothesis is the characteristic of deleteriousness, which has never been proven in either aging neurons or in the heart. There seems to be little doubt that enzymatic defects of the neuronal degradative mechanism can occur in relation to lipid breakdown and in some of these cases dying neurons will contain excessive amounts of lipofuscin (Gonatas et al., 1968; Zeman, 1971). Increased lipofuscin has also been demonstrated in neurons targeted for death in Creutzfeldt-Jakob disease (Freide and DeJong, 1964; Torack, 1969) but this seems to be a secondary response to cell injury and, in itself, is not the cause of cell death. The unresolved question is whether pigment accumulation in aging neurons represents some type of neuronal ceroid lipofuschinosis, a response to some form of chronic cell injury, or merely an aggregate related to time without any pathogenetic implication.

A rational approach to this problem again seems to be whether it is a prominent component of neurons in those locations that are particularly susceptible to aging depletion. A most important consideration is that the neurons of the inferior olive aggregate pigment very early in childhood, and demonstrate prominent lipofuscin throughout life, yet both Moatamed (1966) and Monagle and Brody (1971) have shown no loss of neurons in this structure with age. Conversely, Purkinje cells, which are recognized to be depleted with age, never show prominent lipofuscin (Ellis, 1919). Among cortical areas, there is no indication of unusual lipofuscin aggregates in the superior temporal gyrus although in all areas of cortex lipofuscin is more conspicuous in larger neurons. So, a definitive role of lipofuscin in the lethal processes of aging has not been demonstrated. At this time it is most appropriate to agree with Toth (1968) who concludes, "It appears that the most valuable further contributions will be those that address themselves to the effects of lipofuscin accumulation."

Abnormalities of the Peripheral Neuron

Most of the interest in neuronal aging has been directed at the cell body but age-related changes have been described in the peripheral parts of these cells. Neuroaxonal dystrophy (Sung, 1965), loss of dendrites (Sheibel et al., 1975, 1976) and a loss of synapses (Bondareff and Geinisman, 1976) have all been described in aging and their occurrence could be an indication that the initial cellular injury is not occurring centrally. The decrease in axonal transport recently reported by Geinisman et al. (1977) is quite consistent with this concept. Another aspect of the same problem may be the alteration of the extracellular compartment, which has been described by Bondareff and Lin-Liu (1977). Cragg (1975) was unable to find synaptic changes in aging human cortex but the recognition that they occur in SP seems to indicate some degree of abnormality. Abnormal levels of transmitter substances in dementia (Bowen et al., 1976) may be another manifestation of peripheral neuron dysfunction. There is a great need to expand these preliminary indications of disorder in the peripheral neuron.

A summary of the pathologic characteristics of aging in the brain reveals a striking paucity of definitive information.

1. Brain atrophy is not an inevitable consequence of aging. Rather, it is a process that predominantly affects male brains of heavy weight. Female brains suffer less and minimum-weight brains appear to be spared.

2. There is unquestionable neuronal loss that is age-related but this does not appear to be a random process. Distinctly variable susceptibility is probably best demonstrated in the cerebellar pathway where as many as half the Purkinje cells may die, but the cell loss is less evident in the dentate nucleus and absent in the inferior olive.
3. There is no direct correlation between the occurrence of NF, GVD, SP, and neuron loss.
4. The relationship between lipofuscin and neuron death has not been proven and existing data indicate that an inverse relationship may exist, since pigment-laden cells in the inferior olive survive but lipofuscin-impoverished Purkinje cells die.
5. Peripheral injury involving axons, dendrites, and synapses may offer better opportunities for research than continued study of cell bodies.

Epidemiology of Mental Aging

The frustrating search to establish an objective determinant of diminished mental competence in the elderly population cannot dispel the widespread recognition that achievement in any form decreases after the age of 65 (Korenchevsky, 1965). The elusive factor appears to be highly individual and a product of intrinsic biologic decay plus a variety of socioeconomically related extrinsic influences. A more complete definition of this problem is hindered by limited knowledge of the potential for achievement of individual change that can be correlated with longevity. The first question involves effectiveness of an aging society and the second point is relevant to a longitudinal survey of aging.

Cross-Sectional Survey of Effectiveness

Although the majority of geriatric research is directed toward the problems of aging, another aspect of the problem is afforded by a study of normal old people. This approach has been used by the various surveys that have assayed the numerous factors involved in longevity. These studies have revealed distinctive physiologic and social conditions that appear to have relevance for an extension of the life span (Palmore, 1971). Obviously mental health is one such factor, for the presence of a dementing syndrome is accepted by all as a factor that shortens survival. We have noted previously that the best predictor of this disorder is an evaluation of effectiveness devised by Blessed et al. (1968). If diminished effectiveness has this relationship to dementia, it seems important to know whether a similar occurrence is present in aging, particularly in very old people.

A survey of this problem has been undertaken by a series of interviews with 125 individuals over the age of 65 at four different socioeconomic levels. Part of this population is derived from the GM survey (Sect. 4), which has been supplemented with similar interviews in three lower socioeconomic groups. TG comprises a less expensive condominium arrangement similar to GM. CH is a retirement apartment complex built with Teamster funds and is designed to be within the economic limits of a union pension fund. MCEP is a community-sponsored day center to which anyone come for social and recreational activity. No travel assistance is provided for the people who attend.

In each case an interview lasting an hour is used to evaluate effectiveness based on the scale of Blessed et al. (1968). All of these people have zero ratings on this scale, so three additional levels of activity have been included. The first is a work category in which the individual continues gainful employment of a nature identical or similar to that which had been performed prior to 65. "Community affairs" includes any regularly scheduled participation in organized charitable work but which does not yield financial benefit. Gainful employment and community affairs are considered useful activities. Social and recreational activities (pleasurable) have not been separated or further qualified because in each socioeconomic group, distinctive functions and opportunities are present which preclude overall comparisons.

The evaluation of defects was entirely by means of conversation and no attempt was made for objective analysis. Furthermore there was no attempt to determine a degree of disability; it was simply recorded as being present. Sensory defects included or auditory problems. Physical defects included any general bodily disturbance, of which arthritis and cardiovascular problems were most common. The mental difficulties were predominantly related to benign memory loss; however, difficulties with cognition and calculations were also noted.

The diversity of these groups is reflected in the level of educational achievement but not in activties (Table 8.4). An analysis of participation levels within the various socioeconomic groups fails to reveal striking differences except for CH. The extraordinarily high work effort is a reflection both of the relatively young age (none over 76) and the peculiar orientation of the residence that is self-governing. When useful activity (work and community affairs) is combined, there is no difference between the highest (GM) and the lowest (MCEP) socioeconomic level.

Table 8.4. Relationship between activities and socioeconomic status in a normal aging population

Location	Number	Education			Activities							
		Col-lege	High Sch.	Grade Sch.	Work		Community affairs		Work and community affairs		Social and recreational	
					No.	%	No.	%	No.	%	No.	%
G.M.	66	39	27	0	9	13.6	15	22.7	24	36.4	45	68.2
T.G.	18	5	11	2	2	11.1	7	18.0	9	50.0	18	100.0
C.H.	13	1	12	0	12	92.3	–	–	12	92.3	11	91.6
MCEP	28	2	8	18	6	21.4	3	10.7	9	32.1	26	92.9

The age or the entire group is quite different from that of the general population in that it includes fewer people under 70 and more over 89 (Table 8.5). This emphasis on older subjects was intentional, particularly with regard to the nonagenarians, who were actively recruited. The working status of the entire population seems to be maintained favorably until age 79. Participation in community charitable affairs is continued at least 5 years longer and, especially in the 80–84-year-old groups, seems to be enhanced by an influx from the working segment. Activities related to social affairs and recreation

Table 8.5. Relationship of activities to age in a normal population over 65

Age	Number	Work		Community affairs		Social and rexreational	
		No.	%	No.	%	No.	%
65–69	12	4	33.3	2	16.7	11	96.5
70–74	29	13	44.8	6	20.6	28	96.5
75–79	27	8	29.6	6	22.2	18	66.7
80–84	23	2	8.7	7	30.4	17	73.9
85–89	11	2	19.2	2	19.2	8	72.8
90+	23	2	8.7	2	8.7	18	78.3
Total	125	29	23.2	25	20.0	100	80.0
90+	23	2	8.7	2	8.7	18	78.3

are continued at a significant level even by the nonagernarians. In this group, the preservation of pleasurable but not useful activity seems to indicate that aging reduces but does not eliminate the possibility of effective behavior.

Several investigators (Granick and Patterson, 1971; Pfeiffer, 1971) have emphasized the influence of education and higher socioeconomic status upon longevity. This is quite evident in the current survey (Table 8.6). The most impressive support for this contention is afforded by the number of 90-year-olds at GM, where they form 15.5% of that group. The local medical service of that group must also be considered to be an important factor in this amazing survival.

Table 8.6. Relationship between socioeconomic status and longevity

Age	GM		TG		CH		MCEP	
	No.	%	No.	%	No.	%	No.	%
65–69	0		1	5.5	4	30.8	7	25.0
70–74	4	6.1	4	22.2	8	61.5	13	46.4
75–79	13	19.7	8	44.4	1	7.7	5	17.9
80–84	19	28.8	3	16.7			1	3.6
85–89	9	13.6	1	5.5			1	3.6
90+	21	31.8	1	5.5			1	3.6

The effect of the various defects upon useful activity is somewhat difficult to evaluate from this data (Table 8.7). The 30% incidence of physical defects at age 75–79 may be very important in the reduction of the work force at this time (Table 8.5). The increasing incidence of all sensory, physical and mental defects is probably the determinant in the decreasing participation in community affairs after 85. The most interesting aspect seems to involve the mental problems. Twenty percent of the population even at age 90 do not admit to any memory loss or difficulty with calculations. The maintenance of mental function may be the chief reason why social functions are maintained, since both physical and sensory defects continue to increase.

Table 8.7. Relationship between age and physical or mental handicap in a normal aging population

Age	Sensory defect		Physical defect		Mental defect	
	No.	%	No.	%	No.	%
65–69	0	0	1	8.3	3	25.0
70–74	1	3.4	7	24.1	14	48.3
75–79	2	7.4	8	29.6	14	51.9
80–84	3	13.0	9	39.1	18	78.3
85–89	2	18.0	4	36.4	7	63.6
90+	5	21.7	11	47.8	18	78.3

The results of this survey do not support any contention of age-induced mental decay, as suggested by Foulds and Raven (1948), which should have been most evident in the group of 90-year-olds. Indeed a plateau occurs about the age of 85 in the incidence of mental defects and the decline of effective behavior. Although the total sample is small, the nonagenarian segment is equivalent to that ordinarily found in a population of 850 persons. Therefore the lack of progression of mental problems seems valid and must mean that these changes are age related and not due to age itself.

Longitudinal Survey of Aging

A most important addition to the study of mental aging is the sequential study of an elderly population. The comparison of old and young age groups during a limited period of examination (cross-sectional surveys) is considered to be nonvalid because cultural differences may be discriminating against the elderly. Repetitive testing of the same group of subjects (longitudinal survey) has been devised to eliminate this objection since the basis for comparison is internal, i.e., with the previous status of the individual subject. The advantages of longitudinal testing have been enumerated by Palmore (1974):

> Each panel member can be used as his own control, consistent trends can be distinguished from temporary fluctuations, errors due to retrospective distortion are minimized, early warning signs of disease or death can be studied, cohort differences can be distinguished from age changes, and the effects of one kind of change on another change at a later period can be studied.

Both Botwinnick and Arenberg (1976) and Schaie (1967) have expressed concern about the interpretation of these studies but certain conclusions regarding intelligence and longevity appear worthy of consideration. There seems to be little criticism about retrospective analysis of the various clinical and testing data in order to appreciate their predictive value for disease and death. It seems reasonable to believe that more subtle abnormalities should have enhanced recognition through such an exercise.

The organization of longitudinal study is relatively recent, but since a cross-sectional study can be converted into a longitudinal survey by the process of reexamination, the oldest study actually dates back to 1919 (Owens, 1966). Since that time several surveys have been conducted and a review of the major findings appears to be indicated in order to appreciate the actual value of this work.

Summary of Longitudinal Surveys

1. Survey of Iowa St. freshmen, 1919–1961 (Owens, 1966).
   At Iowa St. University, 127 freshmen took the Army Alpha Intelligence test in 1919 as part of their college entrance examination. They were retested in 1950 and in 1960, at which time 96 subjects were available.
2. New England study, 1958–1966 (Rhudick and Gordon, 1973).
   In an age center, 232 domiciled members, average age 72.6, were given the WAIS test and retested 1–8 years later at an average age of 76.2.
3. Duke longitudinal survey, 1955–1973 (Normal Aging II, 1974).
   From the domiciliary population of Durham, N.C., 271 persons were selected between the ages of 60–90. They were tested originally with the WAIS and retested every 3–4 years until 1965, then every 2 years until 1972. In 1973 all survivors were tested for the eighth time. Intelligence tests were supplemented with EEG, blood flow assay, and serum protein levels.
4. N.Y. State Psychiatric Institute study of senescent twins, 1947–1967 (Blum et al., 1973).
   Two hundred and sixty-eight senescent twins, mean age 69.7, were evaluated using five Wechsler subtests (similarities, digits forward, digits backward, digit symbol substitution, and block design), a local paper and pencil tapping test, and the vocabulary list 1 of Sanford-Binet. Retesting of 73 subjects occurred in 1967.
5. North German survey, 1956–1962 (Riegel et al., 1967).
   A Hamburg WAIS was originally given to 380 normal adults 55+ years old (average age 79.0). Five years later, 202 were available for retesting.
6. VA Hospital Bath, N.Y., 1952–1963 (Berkowitz, 1965).
   The WAIS test was taken by 184 VA domiciliary males at an average age of 56. They were retested 5 or more years later at an average age of 65. A follow-up survey occurred 48 months after the second testing in order to determine survival.
7. NIH study, 1955–1968 (Human Aging II, 1971).
   Forty-seven men with a mean age of 71 (65–91) were subject to extensive medical, psychiatric, and psychological testing in 1955. Follow-up examination occurred in 1961–62 and in 1967–68. Of the original group, 23 were alive for the last testing and 19 participated in the examination. The original subjects were separated into 2 groups. Group 1 had no asymptomatic disease; group 2 had asymptomatic cardiovascular disease, i.e., hypertension. EEG and blood flow assay were included.
8. Baltimore longitudinal study, Stone and Norris (1966).
   463 men living in the Washington D.C. area, of whom 151 were older than 60. The participants were given a medical examination and the Chicago activity and attitude inventory every 19 months.

Psychological Test of Intelligence

The most impressive information, which has now been corroborated by several groups (Riegel et al., 1966; Blum et al., 1973), is that most subtest performance actually improves with age; the only exceptions are those that relate to some aspects of performance, i.e., digit symbol. This is in startling contrast to the unequal but general decline of all subtests revealed by cross-sectional studies. This discrepancy has been studied most extensively by Schaie (1970), who compares the varying results of the two methodologies in Table 8.8.

Table 8.8. Comparison of inferences drawn from cross-sectional longitudinal and short-term longitudinal studies (after Schaie, 1970)

Variable	Cross-sectional	Longitudinal	Short-term longitudinal
Verbal meaning	Sharp decrement from middle adulthood to old age	Modest gain throughout life from young adult plateau	Modest decrement from young adult plateau; increment in successive cohorts reaching asymptote
Space	Sharp decrement from young adult peak to old age	Modest decrement from adult plateau	Almost no decrement until advanced age; steep positive cohort gradient is reaching asymptote
Reasoning	Sharp decrement from young adult peak to old age	Modest gain from young adult plateau till od age	Modest decrement from middle adulthood to old age; positively accelerating cohort gradient
Number	Modest gain and loss before and subsequent to midlife plateau	Modest gain from early adulthood to plateau at advanced age	Very modest decrement from plateau in middle adulthood; positively accelerated cohort gradient
Word fluency	Moderate decrement from plateau extending over major portion of adulthood	Moderate gains from young adult levels	Sharp decrements from young adult levels; steep decrements for successive cohorts

The absence of predicted decline and in some cases actual improvement in verbal performance prompted a reevaluation of the surviving subjects. Many investigators, particularly Riegel et al. (1967), have observed that the nature of the cohort is constantly changing due to the death of biologically less viable individuals. This means that the survivors who are available for retesting become increasingly a group of supernormals. Therefore aging effects that are determined by average test or rating scores are considered to be only partially valid. However, Botwinnick (1973) points out that the original group would not be strictly comparable, even if it were intact, since other factors such as practice incident to second testing and motivation would be different.

Curiously there are very few data on individual performance in repetitive tests. Instead most of the information is presented as repetitive mean or average performance scales. The New England survey (Rhudick and Gordon, 1973) has taken particular note of individual variation and the N.Y. State Psychiatric Institute survey (Blum et al., 1970) has recognized similar inconsistency with mean performance. The degree of variation can be seen in the evaluation of the 19 survivors of the NIH study (Table 8.8). A decline of 24 points in the intelligence test score by two subjects was almost offset by a surprising gain of 16 points by another person. Most amazing is that the latter occurred in an individual who ranked 14th even after this tremendous increase (Patterson et al., 1971). This seems to belie the contention that the poor initial performers deteriorate most.

Psychometrics as Determinants of Longevity

In cross-sectional surveys, poor performance in psychological testing has been widely interpreted as being detrimental to longevity. An adverse prognostic indication in longitudinal testing has been advocated by Berkowitz (1965) but his "imminence of death factor" seems to have self-destructed. The evaluation of these predictors of death by Palmore (1974) reveals that only performance IQ in women over the age of 70 has significance in this regard.

Somewhat surprisingly, several surveys have concluded that certain aspects of behavior have importance for survival. In 1966, Stone and Norris maintained that their group of mobile elderly subjects up to age 90 was characterized by a rentention of social activities and attitudes. A similar thought was expressed by Granick and Patterson (1971) who considered disorganization of behavior (along with cigarette smoking) as the most effective predictors of decreased longevity. A correlation between behavioral rigidity and early death was also proposed by Riegel et al. (1967).

Biologic Factors of Longevity

An influence of bodily health upon survival has been evaluated seriously only by the Duke survey and the NIH study and both agree that general health is more important than mental health. Pritchard (1967) indicated this relationship in his study of previous hospitalization and longevity. Amont the biologic factors cigarette smoking and cardiovascular diesease (Granick and Patterson, 1971; Palmore, 1974) seem to be most important. Another interesting conclusion is that decline in psychological testing can be correlated with cardiovascular disease in general (Granick and Patterson, 1971; Palmore, 1974) and hypertension in particular (Wilkie and Eisdorfer, 1971).

Conclusions

A most tragic circumstance is the dearth of anatomic study of the brain or other organs in these longitudinal studies. In 20 years, the Duke study has not published a single report of a pathologic examination on one of its subjects. The more serious effort to correlate organic brain disease with the other aspects of the study is present in the NIH survey. Indeed there are 4 of the 19 survivors who are labeled "chronic brain syndrome" and each of them had a decline of 16 or more points in test performance (Table 8.9). Unfortunately we learn nothing more about the nature of this decline and its relationship to aging. There are also no pathologic data in this report.

The conclusions of these surveys are diverse and on occasion contradictory, yet certain concepts appear to be possible.

1. Previous reports of overall intellectual decline in aging from cross-sectional surveys are not corroborated by longitudinal studies. Some decay in performance occurs but verbal ability may remain intact or even improve.
2. Measures of behavior may be more important than tests of verbal ability and performance in the determination of longevity. Individual variation in testing of verbal ability and performance is considerable and high initial testing remains a questionable factor in retention of intelligence and survival.
3. The primary determinants of longevity are not initial mental ability but physical disease.
4. There is no aspect of mental aging that can be used to predict dementia.

Table 8.9. Results of longitudinal psychometrics in the survivors of the NIH study (Granick and Patterson, 1971).

Subject number and name		Age t_3	Change of test score t_1 to t_3	Rank of test score t_3
6	Crabtree	84	$- >24$	19
51	Dooley	81	$- 24$	9
18	Everett	78	$- 17$	13
23	Smith	85	$- 16$	18
58	Moran	81	$- 16$	12
56	Bryant	80	$- 15$	7
42	McLure	79	$- 12$	15
54	Lewis	83	$- 11$	5
15	Hyatt	87	$- 8$	10
8	Wozny	83	$- 6$	16
47	Jones	76	$- 4$	3
20	Gottlieb	85	$- 2$	8
9	Dixon	79	0	17
59	Ginsburg	84	$+ 1$	4
27	Tudor	77	$+ 2$	6
55	Postik	75	$+ 7$	1
7	Murray	79	$+ 10$	11
22	Lehigh	81	$+ 11$	2
14	Rhine	80	$+ 16$	14

t_1, initial psychometric examination; t_3, third psychometric examination.

Summary of Mental Aging

There seems to be no aspect of brain function that has been demonstrated to decline with age in a linear manner comparable to mean brain weight. Memory loss is the most common mental defect in aging, yet there is no evidence to indicate that everyone will have this problem at some age or that the usual memory loss becomes more severe with longevity. Only Kral has described a malignant form of memory defect and even this was used as an indicator of reduced survival, not of dementia. The decline of cognitive function has been so confused by the complexities of psychometric testing and by the results of longitudinal studies that the nature of this change, much less its significance, cannot be determined at this time.

There is some evidence that reveals that effective behavior deteriorates with age and that it is a useful indicator of diminished longevity. There is little doubt that psychiatric disorders are very prevalent over 65. The similarity of these disorders to those occurring before 65 and the lack of progression associated with increasing age are strong arguments that brain weight loss is not a factor in their evolution. Rather, their increased incidence is attributable to the stressful emotional and socioeconomic circumstances that frequently occur in elderly life. Perhaps the converse statement would be more correct: that effective behavior in survivors appears to continue indefinitely.

The EEG shows several abnormalities that are present in aged individuals. Their unpredictable occurrence, the lack of continuity, and progressive severity, and the absence of predictive value belie any consideration that these changes are a valid marker of age. Sensory evoked potentials may have greater significance but additional study is needed to prove this contention. Blood flow studies have yielded no alteration correlative to age.

There seems to be little doubt that mean brain weight declines in a linear fashion concurrent with age. However the disparity between male and female weight loss and the realization that minimal brain weight is not altered by age indicates that this is not an inevitable companion of longevity. The cause of the weight loss is undeniably a decrease in the neuronal population and in quantitative assays of neurons very distinct patterns of nerve cell loss have been demonstrated. It is quite important to recognize that some nuclear groups such as the inferior olive show no neuronal decrement with age. A fair conclusion is that the neuronal loss is the result of a selective mechanism, which can occur as early as 25 but in some cases does not operate.

The pathologic correlates of neuron loss are inconclusive. The principal nerve cell changes that have been related to the aging mechanism are not located predominantly in the areas of greatest cell loss. The relationship between lipofuscin and neuron fallout among Purkinje cells and the inferior olive is actually inverse. The best correlation between plaques and cell loss occurs in the temporal lobe but a comparison between frontal and occipital lobes again reveals an inverse relationship.

The longitudinal studies have contradicted the intellectual decline that has been observed in cross-sectional surveys. Verbal decline is not evident and only some aspects of performance deteriorate in repetitive testing. The other chief value of these studies involves the evaluation of various factors in longevity, which reveals that general physical factors appear to be much more important than mental ability.

It seems evident that any concept of mental aging predicates nerve cell death and that this loss of cells is linked with a variety of functional, chemical, and structural defects. However, time is a most uniform determinant and without similar uniformity any brain change cannot be considered to be only time dependent. Indeed it is a lack of consistency that characterizes all of the supposed markers of the aging process. When new criteria of aging are established, they may have more relevance for dementia.

References

Adler, W.H. (1974): An auto-immune theory of aging. In: Theoretical Aspects of Aging. Rockstein, M. (ed.). New York: Academic Press

Adler, W.H., Takiguchi, T., Smith, R.T. (1971): Effect of age upon primary alloantigen recognition by mouse spleen cells. J. Immunol. 107, 1357–1362

Adrian, E.D., Matthews, B.H.C. (1934): The Berger rhythm; potential changes from the occipital lobes in man. Brain 57, 355–384

Appel, F.W., Appel, E.M. (1942): Intracranial variation in the weight of the human brain. Hum. Biol. 14, 235–250

Baer, P.E. (1972): Cognitive changes in aging. In: Aging and the Brain. Gaitz, C.M. (ed.). New York: Plenum

Ball, M.J. (1976): Neurofibrillary tangles and the pathogenesis of dementia: A quantitative study. Neuropathol. Appl. Neurobiol. 2, 395–410

Bender, A.D. (1970): The influence of age on the activity of catecholamines and related therapeutic agents. J. Am. Geriat. Soc. 18. 220–232

Bergmann, K. (1972): Personality traits and reactions to the stresses of aging. In: Aging of the Central Nervous System. Biological and Psychological Aspects. Van Praag, H.M., Kalverboer, A.F. (eds.). Haarlem: De Erven F. Bohn, pp. 162–182

Berkowitz, B. (1965): Changes in intellect with age: IV. Changes in achievement and survival in older people. J. Genet. Psychol. 107, 3–14

Blessed, G., Roth, M., Tomlinson, B.E. (1968): The association between quantitative measures of dementia and of senile change in the cerebral grey matter of elderly subjects. Br. J. Psychiatry 114, 797

Blum, J.E., Clark, E.T., Jarvik, L.F. (1973): In: Intellectual Functioning in Adults. Jarvik, L.F., Eisdorfer, C., Blum, J.E. (eds.). New York: Springer, pp. 13–19

Blum, J.E., Jarvik, L.F., Clark, E.T. (1970): Rate of change on selective tests of intelligence: A twenty-year longitudinal study of aging. J. Gerontol. 25, 171–176

Bock, E., Jorgensen, O.S., Dittman, L., Eng, L.F. (1975): Determination of brain specific antigens in short term cultivated rat astroglial cells and in rat synaptosomes. J. Neurochem. 25, 867–870

Bondareff, W., Geinisman, Y. (1976): Loss of synapses in the dentate gyrus of the senescent rat. Am. J. Anat. 145, 129–136

Bondareff, W., Lin-Liu, S. (1977): Age-related change in the neuronal microenvironment: Penetration of ruthenium red into extracellular space of brain in young adult and senescent rats. Am. J. Anat. 148, 57–64

Botwinnick, J. (1967): Cognitive Processes in Maturity and Old Age. New York: Springer

Botwinnick, J. (1973): Aging and Behavior. New York: Springer

Botwinnick, J., Arenberg, D. (1976): Disparate time spans in sequential studies of aging. Exp. Aging Res. 2, 55–61

Botwinnick, J., Storandt, M. (1974): Memory, Related Functions, and Age. Springfield: C.C. Thomas

Brody, H. (1955): Organization of the cerebral cortex. III. A study of aging in the human cerebral cortex. J. Comp. Neurol. 102, 511–556

Brody, H. (1970): Structural changes in the aging nervous system. Interdiscipl. Topics Gerontol. 7, 9–21

Buckley, C.E., Buckley, E.G., Dorsey, F.C. (1974): Longitudinal changes in serum immunoglobulin levels in older humans. Fed. Proc. 33, 2036–2039

Burger, M. (1954): Altern und Krankheit. Leipzig: Georg Thieme

Busse, E.W., Obrist, W.D. (1963): Significance of focal electroencephalic changes in the elderly. Postgrad. Med. 34, 179–182

Busse, E.W., Wang, H.S. (1965): The value of electroencephalography in geriatrics. Geriatrics 20, 906–924

Campbell, B.A., Spear, N.E. (1972): Ontogeny of memory. Psychol. Rev. 79, 215–236

Ciompi, L. (1969): Followup studies on the evolution of former neurotic and depressive states in old age. J. Geriatr. Psychiatry 3, 90–106

Colon, E.J. (1972): Quantitative cytoarchitectonics of the human cerebral cortex in schizophrenic dementia. Acta Neuropath. 20, 1–10

Corso, J.F. (1975): Sensory processes in man during maturity and senescence. In: Neurobiology of Aging. Ordy, J.M., Brizzee, K.R. (eds.). New York: Plenum, pp. 119–143

Couch, H.N. (1959): Cicero on the Art of Growing Old. Ilfracombe: A.H. Stockwell

Cragg, B.G. (1975): The density of synapses and neurons in normal, mentally defective and aging human brains. Brain 98, 81–90

Critchley, M. (1931): The neurology of old age. Lancet 1119–1127

Dastur, D.K., Lane, M.H., Hansen, D.B., Kety, S.S., Butler, R.N., Perlin, S., Sokoloff, L. (1963): Effects of aging on cerebral circulation and metabolism in man. In: Human Aging. A Biological and Behavioral Study. Birren, J., et al. (eds.). Bethesda: U.S. Govt. Printing Office

Dustman, R.E., Beck, E.C. (1969): The effects of maturation and aging on the wave form of visually evoked potentials. Electroencephal. Clin. Neurophysiol. 26, 2–11

Ellingson, R.J. (1966): Relationship between EEG and test intelligence: A commentary. Psychol. Bull. 65, 91–98

Ellis, R.S. (1919): A preliminary quantitative study of the Purkinje cells in normal, subnormal, and senescent human cerebella, with some notes on functional localization. J. Comp. Neurol. 30, 229–252

Ellis, R.S. (1920): Norms for some structural changes in the human cerebellum from birth to old age. J. Comp. Neurol. 32, 1–33

Fazekas, J.F., Alman, R.W., Bessman, A.N. (1952): Cerebral physiology of the aged. Am. J. Med. Sci. 223, 245–257

Fazekas, J.R., Kleh, J., Witkin, L. (1953): Cerebral hemodynamics and metabolism in subjects over 90 years of age. J. Am. Geriatr. Assoc. 1, 836–839

Foulds, G.A., Raven, J.C. (1948): Normal changes in the mental abilities of adults as age advances. J. Ment. Sci. 94, 133–142

Friede, R.L., DeJong, R.N. (1964): Neuronal enzymatic failure in Creutzfeldt-Jakob disease. Arch. Neurol. 10, 181–185

Gardner, E. (1940): Decrease in human neurons with age. Anat. Rec. 77, 529–536

Geinisman, Y., Bondareff, W., Telser, A. (1977): Diminished axonal transport of glycoprotein in the senescent rat brain. Mech. Aging Develop. 6, 363–378

Gold, P.E., McGaugh, J.L. (1975): Changes in learning during aging. In: Neurobiology of Aging. Ordy, J.M., Brizzee, K.E. (eds.). New York: Plenum Press, pp. 145–148

Goldfarb, A.I. (1975): Memory and aging. In: The Physiology and Pathology of Human Aging. Goldman, R., Rockstein, M. (eds.). New York: Academic Press, pp. 149–186

Granick, S., Patterson, R.D. (1971): Human Aging II. An Eleven-year Followup Biomedical and Behavioral Study. Rockville: DHEW Publ. # 71-9037, pp. 129–137

Haferkamp, O., Schlettwein-Gsell, D., Schwick, H.G., Storiko, K. (1966): Serum protein in an aging population with particular reference to evaluation of immune globulins and antibodies. Gerontology 12, 30–38

Hall, T.C., Miller, A.K.H., Corsellis, J.A.N. (1975): Variations in the human Purkinje cell population according to age and sex. Neuropathol. Appl. Neurobiol. 1, 267–292

Hamilton, G.V. (1938): Changes in personality and psychosexual phenomena with age. In: Cowdry EV. Problems of Aging. Biological and Medical Aspects. Baltimore: Williams and Wilkins, pp. 459–482

Henderson, G., Tomlinson, B.E., Weightman, D. (1975): Cell counts in the human cerebral cortex using a traditional and an automatic method. J. Neurol. Sci. 25, 129–144

Heron, A., Chown, S. (1967): Age and Function. Boston: Little, Brown

Hoch-Ligeti, C. (1963): Effect of aging on the central nervous system. J. Am. Geriatr. Soc. 11, 403–408

Hoedt-Rasmussen, K. (1965): Regional cerebral blood flow in man measured externally following nitra-arterial administration of ^{85}Kr or ^{133}Xc dissolved in saline. Acta Neurol. Scand. 41, (Suppl. 14), 65–68

Hubbard, O., Sunde, D., Goldensohn, E.S. (1976): The EEG in centanarians. Electroencephal. Clin. Neurophysiol. 40, 407–417

Humphrey, T. (1944): Primitive neurons in the embryonic human central nervous system. J. Comp. Neurol. 81, 24–45

Ingvar, D.H., Baldy-Mouliner, M., Sulg, I., Horman, S. (1965): Regional cerebral blood flow related to EEG. Acta Neurol. Scand. 41 (Suppl. 14), 179–182

Ingvar, D.H., Cronqvist, S., Ekberg, R., Risberg, J., Hoedt-Rasmussen, K. (1965): Normal values of regional cerebral blood flow in man, including flow and weight estimates of gray and white matter. Acta Neurol. Scand. 41 (Suppl. 14), 72–78

Ingvar, D.H., Schwartz, M.S. (1974): Blood flow patterns induced in the dominant hemisphere by speech and adding. Brain 97, 273–288

Jarvik, M.E. (1972): Effects of chemical and physiological treatments on learning and memory. Ann. Rev. Psychol. 23, 453–486

Kay, D.W.K., Beamish, P., Roth, M. (1964): Old age mental disorders in Newcastle upon Tyne. Part II. A study of possible social and medical causes. Br. J. Psychiatry 110, 668–682

Kety, S.S., Schmidt, C.F. (1945): The determination of cerebral blood flow in man by the use of nitrous oxide in low concentrations. Am. J. Physiol. 143, 53–66

Klonoff, H., Kennedy, M. (1965): Memory and perceptual functioning in octogenarians and nonagenerians in the community. J. Gerontol. 20, 328–333

Konigsmark, B.W., Murphy, E.A. (1970): Neuronal populations in the human brain. Nature 228, 1335–1336

Kooi, K.A., Guvener, A.M., Tupper, C.J., Bagchi, B.K. (1964): Electroecephalographic patterns of the temporal region in normal adults. Neurology 14, 1029–1035

Korenchevsky, V. (1961): Physiological and Pathological Aging. New York: Hafner

Kral, V.A. (1962): Senescent forgetfulness: Benign and malignant. Can. Med. Assoc. J. 86, 256–260

Lee, R.G., Blair, R.D.G. (1973): Evolution of EEG and visual evoked response changes in Jakob-Creutzfeldt disease. Electroencephal. Clin. Neurophysiol. 35, 133–142

Libow, L.S., Obrist, W.D., Sokoloff, L. (1971): Cerebral circulatory and electroencephalic changes in elderly man. In: Human Aging II. An Eleven-Year Followup. Biomedical and Behavioral Study. Granich, S., Patterson, R.D. (eds.). Rockvill, DHEW Pub. 71-9037, pp. 41–62

MacKeown, F. (1975): De Senectute. J. R. Coll. Physicians 10, 79–99

Makinodan, T., Perkins, E.H., Chen, M.G. (1971): Immunologic activity of the aged. Adv. Gerontol. Res. 3, 171–198

Maletta, G.J. (1974): Survey Report on the Aging Nervous System. Rockville, DHEW Publication # 74-296

Mankovsky, N., Belonog, R. (1971): Aging of the human nervous system in the electroencephalic aspect. Geriatrics 260, 100

McGaugh, J.L. (1973): Drug facilitation of learning and memory. Ann. Rev. Pharmacol. 13, 229–241

McGaugh, J.L., Herz, M.J. (1972): Memory Consolidation. San Francisco: Albion

Mengoli, G. (1952): The EEG in old age. Electroencephal. Clin. Neurophysiol. 4, 232–233

Mirsky, A.F., Harmon, N. (1974): The problem of attention impairment in aging. In: Survey Report on the Aging Nervous System. Maletta, G.J. (ed.). Rockville, DHEW Publication, 74-296, pp. 187–194

Moatamed, F. (1966): Cell frequencies in the human inferior olivary nuclear complex. J. Comp. Neurol. 128, 109–116

Monagle, R.D., Brody, H. (1971): The effects of age upon the main nucleus of the inferior olive in the human. J. Comp. Neurol. 155, 61–66

Muller, C. (1971): Schizophrenia in advanced senescence. Br. J. Psychiatry 118, 247–248

Mundy-Castle, A. (1951): Theta and beta rhythm in the electroencephalograms of normal adults. Electroencephal. Clin. Neurophysiol. 3, 477–486

Nandy, K., Fritz, R.B., Threatt, J. (1975): Specificity of brain-reactive antibodies in serum of old mice. J. Gerontol. 30, 269–274

Nelson, K., Gellhorn, E. (1958): The influence of age and functional neuropsychiatric disorders on sympathetic and parasympathetic functions. J. Psychosom. Res. 3, 12–26

Netboy, A. (1974): The Salmon. Their Fight for Survival. Boston: Houghton Mifflin

Obrist, W.D. (1963): The electroencephalogram of healthy aged males. In: Human Aging. A Biological and Behavioral Study. Birren, J.E. et al. (eds.). Bethesda: U.S. Govt. Printing Office

Obrist, W.D. (1972): EEG and intellectual function in the aged. Electroencephal. Clin. Neurophysiol. 33, 253

Obrist, W.D., Sokoloff, L., Lassen, N.A., Lane, M.H., Butler, R.N., Feinberg, I. (1963): Relation of EEG to cerebral blood flow and metabolism in old age. Electroenceph. Clin. Neurophysiol. 15, 610–619

Ordy, J.M., Brizzee, K.R. (1975): Neurobiology of Aging. An Interdisciplinary Life-Span Approach. New York: Plenum Press

Owens, W.A. (1966): Age and mental abilities: A second adult follow up. J. Educ. Psychol. 57, 311–325

Palmore, E. (1974): In: Normal Aging II. Durham: Duke Univ. Press, pp. 286–290

Patterson, R.D., Freeman, L.C., Butler, R.N. (1971): Psychiatric aspects of adaptation survival and death. In: Human Aging II. An Eleven-year Followup. Biomedical and Behavioral Study. Granick, S., Patterson, R.D. (eds.). Rockville, DHEW Publ. 71-9036

Pearl, R. (1905): Biometrical studies on man. I. Variation and correlation in brain-weight. Biometrika 4, 13–104

Peress, N.S., Kane, W.C., Aronson, S.M. (1973): Central nervous system findings in a tenth decade autopsy population. Prog. Brain Res. 40, 473–483

Pfeiffer, E. (1971): Physical, psychological, and social correlates of survival in old age. Prediction of life span. Palmore, E., Jeffers, F. (eds.). Lexington: Health Lexington, pp. 223–236

Post, F. (1962): The Significance of Affective Symptoms in Old Age. London: Oxford Univ. Press

Pritchard, J.G. (1967): On the past history. A study of previous hospitalization and its influence on longevity. Gerontol. Clin. 9, 140–148

Rhudick, P.J., Gordon, C. (1973): The age center of New England study. In: Intellectual Functioning in Adults. Jarvik, L.C., Eisdorfer, C., Blum, J.E. (eds.). New York: Springer, pp. 7–12

Riegel, K.F., Riegel, R.M., Meyer, G. (1967): A study of the dropout rates in longitudinal research on aging and the prediction of death. J. Person. Soc. Psychol. 5, 342–348

Roberts-Thomson, I.C., Whittingham, S., Youngchaiyud, U., Mackay, I.R. (1974): Aging, immune response, and mortality. Lancet 2, 368–370

Roth, M. (1955): The natural history of mental disorder in old age. J. Ment. Sci. 101, 281–301

Russell, W.R. (1959): Brain, Memory, Learning. Oxford: Clarendon

Schaie, K.W. (1967): Age changes and age differences. Gerontology 7, 128–132

Schaie, K.W. (1970): A reinterpretation of age related changes in cognitive structure and functioning. In: Life-Span Developmental Psychology. Goulet, L.R., Baltes, P.B. (eds.). New York: Academic Press, pp. 485–507

Scheibel, M.E., Lindsay, R.D., Tomiyasu, U., Scheibel, A.B. (1975): Progressive dendritic changes in aging human cortex. Exp. Neurol. 47, 392–403

Scheibel, M.E., Lindsay, R.D., Tomixasu, U., Scheibel, A.B. (1976): Progressive dendritic changes in the aging human limbic system. Exp. Neurol. 53, 420–430

Shefer, V.F. (1972): Absolute number of neurons and thickness of the cerebral cortex during aging, senile and vascular dementia, and Pick's and Alzheimer's diseases. Zhurnal. Nevropathol. Psikhiatr. Korsak. 72, 1024–1029

Sheridan, F.P., Yeager, C.L., Oliver, W.A., Simon, A. (1955): Electroencephalography as a diagnostic and prognostic and in studying the senescent individual. A preliminary report. J. Gerontol. 10, 53–59

Sherkin, A. (1974): Higher cognitive processes. In: Summary Report on the Aging Nervous System. Maletta, G.J. (ed.). Rockville, DHEW Publ. 74-296, pp. 179–184

Shucard, D.W., Horn, J.L. (1972): Evoked cortical potentials and measurement of human abilities. J. Comp. Physiol. Psychol. 78, 59–68

Stone, J.L., Norris, A.H. (1966): Activities and attitudes of participants in the Baltimore longitudinal study. J. Gerontol. 21, 575–580

Straumanis, J.J., Shagass, C., Schwartz, M. (1965): Visually evoked cerebral response changes associated with chronic brain syndromes and aging. J. Gerontol. 20, 498–506

Strehler, B.L., Mark, D.D., Mildvan, A.S., Gee, M.V. (1959): Rate and magnitude of age pigment accumulation in the human myocardium. J. Gerontol. 14, 430–439

Sung, J.H. (1965): Neuroaxonal dystrophy in aging. Proc. Fifth Int. Cong. Neuropathol. Luthy, F., Bischoff, A. (eds.). Amsterdam: Excerpta Medica, pp. 478–480

Terry, R.D., Fitzgerald, C., Peck, A., Millner, J., Farmer, P. (1977): Cortical cell counts in senile dementia. J. Neuropathol. Exp. Neurol. 36, 633

Threatt, J., Nandy, K., Fritz, R. (1971): Brain-reactive antibodies in serum of old mice demonstrated by immunofluorescence. J. Gerontol. 26, 316–323

Tomlinson, B.E., Blessed, G., Roth, M. (1968): Observations on the brains of non-demented old people. J. Neurol. Sci. 7, 331–356

Torack, R.M. (1969): Ultrastructural and histochemical studies of cortical biopsies in subacute dementia. Acta Neuropathol. 13, 43–55

Toth, S.E. (1968): The origin of lipofuscin age pigments. Exp. Gerontol. 3, 19–30

Visser, S.L., Stam, F.C., VanTilburg, W., Op Den Velde, W., Blom, J.L., De Rijke, W. (1976): Visual evoked response in senile and presenile dementia. Electroencephal. Clin. Neurophysiol. 40, 385–392

Vogel, W., Broverman, D.M. (1966): A reply to "Relationship between EEG and test intelligence: A commentary". Psychol. Bull. 65, 99–109

Walford, R.L. (1965): The general immunology of aging. Adv. Gerontol. Res. 2, 159–204

Walford, R.L. (1969): The Immunologic Theory of Aging. Baltimore: Wilkins and Williams

Wang, H.S., Obrist, W.D., Busse, E.W. (1974): Neurophysiological correlates of intellectual function. In: Normal Aging II. Durham: Duke Univ. Press, pp. 115–126

Warthin, A.S. (1928): The pathology of the aging process. Bull. N.Y. Acad. Med. 4, 1006–1046

Weinberg, H. (1969): Correlation of frequence spectra of averaged visual evoked potentials with verbal intelligence. Nature 224, 813–814

Weksler, M.E., Hutteroth, T.H. (1974): Impaired lymphocyte function in aged humans. J. Clin. Invest. 53, 99–104

Wilkie, F., Eisdorfer, C. (1971): Intelligence and blood pressure in the aged. Science 172, 959

Wilkinson, I.M.S., Bull, J.W.D., DuBoulay, G.H., Marshall, J., Ross Russell, R.W., Symon, L. (1969): Regional blood flow in the normal cerebral hemisphere. J. Neurol. Neurosurg. Psychiatry 32, 367–378

Yakovlev, P.I. (1948): Motility, behavior, and the brain. Stereodynamic organization and neural co-ordinates of behavior. J. Nerv. Ment. Dis. 107, 313–335

Zeman, W. (1971): The neuronal ceroid-lipofuscinosis-Batten-Vogt syndrome: A model for human aging? Adv. Gerontol. Res. 3, 147–170

9. Nature and Cause of Alzheimer's Disease: The Case for Slow Virus Infection

The discovery of lesions in the brain (of dementia) and their classification make, of course, only one step in the determination of their aetiology, but surely a necessary step if any scientific progress is to be made. (Greenfield, 1939.)

The pathologist and the electron microscopist – in spite of the undoubted value of biopsy and the advances in cytochemistry – see only the debris of the battlefield and it is left to the clinician, the neurophysiologist and the chemist to deduce what actually happens in the struggle between the healthy brain and the disturbance (dementia), which affects it. (McMenemey, 1968.)

After 70 years of lesion scrutiny and war correspondence, the etiology of Alzheimer's disease is unknown. (Torack, 1976.)

A most difficult task for nosology is to categorize, as anything other than cryptogenic, a disease that has no distinctive clinical syndrome no predictive diagnostic test, no pathognomicmorphology and no effective treatment. In this bleak situation, a useful exercise would seem to involve a summation of clinical, diagnostic, epidemiologic, and pathologic knowledge in order to identify the involved brain more clearly on a functional, regional, and cellular level. Then, an evaluation of etiology can be based on the potential of various agents to effect these characteristics.

A most important attitude in this approach to Alzheimer's disease (AD) involves amnesia for all preconceived ideas about the basic abnormality of this problem. Since the time of Hughlings Jackson, the expression of dementia has been considered to represent neocortical dysfunction, and indeed cortical dementia appears to be exemplified by Creutzfeldt-Jakob disease (CJD). However, the neocortex is uninvolved in normal pressure hydrocephalus (NPH), which actually appears to be a disease of Yakovlev's entopallium. The recognition of limbic dementia means that a dementing syndrome can be the consequence of disorder in the mesopallium of the triune brain. Therefore, the characterization of AD should be limited only by the absence of vascular disease and aging as etiologic agents.

Nature of AD

Clinical Indicators

The most early clinical symptoms seem to be a loss of past memory coupled with disorientation for time and place. Both appear to be facets of impaired information processing, which has been primarily localized to the temporal lobe (Victor, 1969). RNA has been proposed as a chemical substrate for this process, but altered RNA metabolism is not present and RNA treatment is ineffective. The early stages of dementia frequently have affective symptoms of depression. anxiety, paranoia, and excitement plus schizophrenia. An etiologic relationship with AD has been considered on the basis of incidence, but stronger support of this contention accrues from the changing pattern of responsiveness to psychoactive drug therapy. The initial effectiveness of these drugs is similar to functional psychosyndromes and it seems to indicate that transmitter imbalance is an early feature of AD.

The development of agnosia, alexia, and apraxia apparently means that neocortical involvement is occurring during the intermediate phases of this disease. These "focal symptoms" were once believed to be characteristic of early age onset (presenile dementia) and they constituted a major clinical criterion for distinction from senile dementia. The realization that this contention is not valid was a major factor in the abolition of the age distinction between senile and presenile dementia. The focal symptoms may still indicate more extensive disease, but seem to have no other etiologic significance.

The terminal pattern of Klüver-Bucy syndrome again appears to link the disease with the temporal lobe, particularly that part belonging to the mesopallium (limbic system). The syndrome has been characterized in animals that have had surgical extirpation of this part of the brain. Similar clinical symptoms have been described in limbic encephalitis, especially herpes simplex.

Progression of mental decay is the final topic in need of reconsideration. Episodic exacerbation, even without focal neurologic signs or symptoms, has been considered an indication of arteriosclerotic dementia. However 25% of all diagnosed vascular dementia cannot be confirmed by the presence of infarcts on pathologic examination. These are largely patients without focal neurologic abnormality. Therefore, episodic exacerbation alone should be considered AD rather than arteriosclerotic dementia. However, this creates a problem since the linear course of AD is believed to be the result of accelerated aging. This means that episodic AD is not consistent with either a vascular or aging etiology.

Diagnostic Criteria

A most disappointing occurrence has been the realization that psychological tests of memory, verbal ability, and performance are not useful in early diagnosis or in prediction of AD. However, these measures are generally designed to measure neocortical function so their failure should be an indication that this is not primarily a neocortical problem. The only psychological evaluation, which appears to have merit for pathology, is the test of effective behavior devised by Blessed et al. (1968). It seems noteworthy that effective behavior is the only aspect of intellectual assays that has been considered to have predictive value for longevity by the NIH study. Control of behavior has been considered to be a function of the limbic system ever since the findings of Papez (1937).

The lack of consistent and progressive changes in EEG of old and demented people seems to emphasize the results of psychometrics. There is no question about the accuracy of sensitivity of the instrument to detect focal or diffuse dysfunction of cortical neurons in epilepsy and other cortical neuronal degenerative disease. Therefore, the realization of ineffectiveness of the EEG in dementia seems to indicate that the abnormality is not at that site. This idea is reinforced by the realization that the chief value of EEG in dementia is in CJD, where cortical involvement is obvious.

Equally frustrating is the failure of cortical biopsy to be more useful not only as a diagnostic tool but especially as a means of determining the chemical and morphologic substrate of AD. To be sure, electron microscopy has extended our knowledge of senile plaques (SP) and neurofibrillary tangles (NF). But the inability of neurochemistry to reveal anything more distinctive than the acid polysaccharides of amyloid is absolutely amazing. It seems unlikely that a significant chemical disorder could not be detected or at least suspected by modern neurochemistry. A more reasonable approach is that perhaps we have been looking in the wrong place.

Epidemiology

The epidemiologic data are characterized by a wide variation in the incidence of AD. Unfortunately, this image is blurred largely as a consequence of the lack of uniformity involving the cohort population, the methods of acquiring data, and the diagnostic criteria. Just the realization that 25% of vascular dementia is AD is sufficient proof that new studies of epidemiology are absolutely necessary. Nevertheless, some relevant information does appear in existing studies.

The association of AD with time reveals that it is age related, but not age dependent. It is unfortunate that so many surveys have not broken down the over-65 population completely, but the Stockholm survey, the GM survey, and the autopsy studies support the contention that nonagenarians do not have more dementia than younger age groups between 75 and 89 (Sect. 4). In reality, they seem to have less. The mental viability of the aging population is revealed in longitudinal surveys by the lack of decline in most areas of verbal ability and performance. These 90-year-olds are also characterized by cerebral blood flow, EEG, and pathologic change that is no different than at age 80. They belie any contention that we will all become demented if we live long enough.

There is a very perplexing aspect to the prevalence studies in that no one seems to believe what they are saying. In Copenhagen, 1.3% of 70-year-olds have senile dementia, but in rural Denmark (Samso) 13.7% of the population aged 70–74 have this problem. In rural Sweden, 22% of the 70–79 age group developed senile psychosis during a 10-year perdiod of study. This seems to be an epidemic of catastrophic proportions, yet the only search for a cause to this problem is the study of Larsson et al. (1963), which investigated genetic influence on AD in Stockholm. Samso has particular attraction, since it is an island and the population would therefore be likely to be even more inbred. Repeat surveys in these rural groups are necessary to confirm earlier findings and to search for genetic and other etiologic factors.

Pathologic Data

There seems to be little doubt that AD results in an increased loss of brain tissue and that this change is at the expense of the neuronal population. The existing quantitative studies of neuron loss indicate that the median temporal lobe, subiculum, and hippocampus is the major site of involvement rather than the neocortex (Shefer, 1972; Ball, 1976; Terry, 1977). The sequence of cellular events leading to this neuronal destruction remains indefinite. Granulovacuolar degeneration is undefined in terms of pathogenetic significance or in relationship to neuronal loss. NF seem to be considered best as a cell body response to distant injury. The evidence for abnormal protein synthesis remains unconfirmed. The major valid indicator of disease seems to be the SP. A most reasonable concept of plaque formation involves some etiologic agent acting focally to disrupt axon flow in distal axons and dendrites, as well as synapses. The dystrophic process causes cytoplasmic organelles, especially neurofilaments, to accumulate, increasing the diameter of these neurites. The mechanism appears to be destructive to these neuronal processes, so that loss of dendrites, axons, and synapses occurs. As these cellular structures break down, their contents including the neurofilaments, are liberated. The neurofilamentous protein and tubulin are antigens that stimulate an immune response in the reticuloendo-thelial system of the brain, resulting in the degradation of the protein and the produc-tion of amyloid. The amyloid is slowly mobilized, so it forms aggregates, which persist in the extracellular space after the cell-destructive phase is completed. Eventually the amyloid also disappears and only the loss of neurites and synapses will be present. Suf-ficient destruction of the peripheral neuron will stimulate a reaction in the cell body, essentially indentical to axon section, which we call an NF.

The formation of amyloid in SP makes the brain the chief producer of this enigmatic material. Paradoxically no one has demonstrated brain amyloid in experimental amyloi-dosis, probably because the blood-brain barrier excludes circulating amyloid precursors. So, the substrate for amyloid seems likely to originate from the brain and neuronal fi-brous proteins appear a most logical choice. Although amyloid production seems to be a secondary reaction, the association between amyloid and immunologic disorders sug-gests that brain immunocompetence is abnormal in AD. Congophilic angiopathy appears to have distinctive amyloid deposition, which may be dependent on a circulating sub-strate and may accompany or even precede the neurite dystrophy. Such amyloid deposi-tion occurs in a hereditary human disease, in aged dogs and monkeys.

Although vascular disease is not a cause of AD, a similar dementing syndrome occurs after multiple brain infarcts have destroyed a mass of tissue varying from 60—412 ml in volume. In smaller volume destruction, the location of these infarcts appears to be criti-cal and they are chiefly in white matter, involving the corpus callosum, the temporal and occipital lobes. Temporal and occipital dysfunction can also result from vertebrobasilar insufficiency and can include a dementing syndrome. The medial temporal lobe and infe-rior occipital lobe are the areas that are chiefly dependent on the posterior circulation.

The concept of AD that emerges from this information is an abnormality of human behavior that is age related and has a hereditary factor. The limbic system, especially the medial temporal lobe, appears to be the target of the disease resulting in a defect that affects the processing of information. The initial cellular disorder involves the peripheral neuron altering neural transmission and resulting in various psychosyndromes. These dis-orders become refractory to treatment as the cellular destruction is more widespread. Collapse of integrated behavior is terminated in many cases by symptoms analogous to surgical resection of the median temporal lobe. The pathologic correlate of the clinical disorder is brain atrophy that is the result of neuron disease. The SP seems to be the chief cellular abnormality relating to this dysfunction. Altered immunocompetence is suggested by the presence of the amyloid in SP.

There are many indications that the dementia of aging is not a single etiologic entity. If some cases of acute confusion terminate as AD, either clinically or pathologically, a whole array of metabolic factors are implicated. Congophilic angiopathy suggests a disorder associated with a generalized immune abnormality. Progressive dementia and NF in chronic lead intoxication links metallic poisoning with the dementing process. A transmissible agent is recognized as the cause of CJD and some cases of CJD have a prolonged clinical course like AD. Therefore, a most reasonable idea is that some agent within these nosologic categories is responsible for the bulk of dementia in the elderly that is represented by typical AD.

Etiologic Potential for AD

Metabolic Disease

This necessarily diffuse category merits consideration from the implied, but unproven, relationship between acute confusional states and chronic organic psychosis. The reversibility of a majority of these disorders suggests a functional abnormality, but the grave prognosis in 50% of hospitalized victims connotes organic disease. The lack of recorded pathologic changes seems to indicate that the usual morphologic correlates of AD are not present. The diverse nature of circumstances leading to acute confusion difies any consideration of regional or specific cellular abnormality. This entity constitutes one of the major frontiers in AD research.

Autoimmune Disease

The participation of the brain in autoimmune reaction has been questioned because of the impermeability of the microcirculation to circulating antibodies and because of the apparent lack of plasma cells to produce local antibodies. However, the evolution of experimental allergic encephalitis (EAE) has demonstrated that myelin proteins are antigenic and that circulating antibodies against these antigens can gain access to the brain. Moreover, a human counterpart to the experimental disease appears to be post-infectious encephalomyelitis. There are several definite ideas of how altered immune mechanisms can lead to neuron death. Burch and Burwell (1965) proposed that a clone of immunocompetent cells has escaped control and produces antibodies causing the death of specific cells. Another concept involves decreased immunocompetence (Nandy, 1975), so that cellular antigens released by normal cycling are not efficiently destroyed. Finally, immunoincompetence has been linked with an expression of virus infection, either endogenous or exogenous (Adler, 1974).

The recent demonstration of brain-reactive antibodies in the sera of aging mice (Nandy, 1973) has stimulated interest not only in an immune mechanism to explain the neuronal loss associated with age, but also the accelerated neuronal death associated with AD. These antibodies are reported to be neuron specific (Nandy et al., 1975) and are not produced by young mice, although they appear capable of binding to neurons in young mice (Nandy, 1975). The antibodies are excluded from the normal aging mouse brain by the blood-brain barrier (Threatt et al., 1971). The antigenicity of tubulin and neurofibrillary protein offer possibilities for the stimulation of neuron-specific antibodies (Schlaepfer, 1976).

Another aspect of immunocompetence may be afforded by the presence of amyloid. In virtue of its occurrence in SP, the brain produces more amyloid than any other organ. The formation of amyloid in plaques has been explained by the availability of fibrous protein substrate following degeneration of dystrophic neurites, yet amyloid does not occur in neuraxonal dystrophy, where even more massive amounts of neurofilaments are occurring. Systemic amyloidosis has been linked with a variety of immunologic disorders, but the precise mechanisms involved in this association are only partially understood (Cohen and Cathcart, 1974). Amyloid formation in the brain is more confused because the brain does not partake in experimental amyloidosis.

The third reason to believe that an immune disorder may be implicated in AD is the early evolution of dementia with plaques and tangles in Down's syndrome (Burger and Vogel, 1973; Ellis et al., 1974). High rate of infection and elevated serum levels of immunoglobulin (Rundle et al., 1971; Dyggve and Clausen, 1970) have led to a belief that altered immunocompetence occurs. However, the elevated serum IgG could be the result not the cause of the infections and the infections may be due to altered leukocyte function (Gregory et al., 1972). The best evidence for an immune abnormality is the decreased responsiveness to phytohemagglutinin by cultured lymphocytes (Agarwal et al., 1970; Nadler et al., 1969). Persistent infection with Australia antigen is also cited as an indication of altered immunity (Hsia et al., 1971).

At this time, definite information regarding immunologic indices of AD is extremely sparse, Behan and Feldman (1970) reported low serum albumin and elevated serum gamma globulins very similar to that found in systemic amyloidosis. A similar pattern of serum proteins was noted by Kalter and Kelly (1975), but Bock et al. (1974) found no specific quantitative changes in either the serum or CSF in patients with dementia but not necessarily AD. It appears important to add that the humoral response described in the serum has no counterpart in the CSF. No one has described significant elevation of either total protein or IgG in AD.

Any conception of AD as autoimmune disease has received very little support in the medical literature. No detectable antibodies could be observed by either Kalter and Kelly (1975) or by Bock et al. (1974) and the preliminary report of antibodies by Tkach and Hokama (1970) has never been confirmed. The lack of antibody detection may be questionable, since the brain antigens were not very specific. The competence of cellular immunity has been confirmed by normal DNA synthesis in mitogen-induced blast-cell transformation and normal thymidine uptake in PHA-stimulated lymphocytes (Kalter and Kelly, 1975). The recent observation that neurofilamentous protein is antigenic (Schlaepfer, 1976) means that the question of autoimmune disease cannot be discarded. This antigenicity, plus the capability to be a substrate for amyloid production, indicate potent immune potential for this protein.

Metallic Intoxication

The neurotoxicity of many heavy metals has been recognized for many years, especially that involving lead (Chisolm, 1970). Peripheral neuropathy, acute encephalopathy and, more recently, chronic encephalopathy have been described clinically and pathologically. Those patients who survive acute encephalopathy develop memory defects and progressive dementia. In these cases, greatest interest is aroused by the demonstration of particular involvement of the hippocampus and by the presence of NF (Niklowitz and Mandybur, 1974). Lead toxicity is well documented in these cases and NF have also been reported in rabbits poisoned with tetraethyl lead.

However, in addition to lead, CNS involvement with dementia can be seen in chronic toxicity due to mercury, arsenic, and thallium (Chisolm, 1970). Methyl mercury poisoning (Minamata disease) has been studied most extensively and focal cortical atrophy, especially of the calcarine cortex, has been demonstrated (Takeuchi et al., 1962). Manganese has been implicated in amyotrophic lateral sclerosis and more recently in Parkinson's disease. Iron and calcium deposits are part of the pathology of Hallervorden-Spatz diesease and two cases of aluminum encephalopathy have been reported. The effects of heavy metals on cell biology are quite widespread, but the emphasis has been upon their effects on membrane permeability or on a variety of enzyme activites chiefly involving energy production.

The argument for aluminum poisoning as the cause of AD is based upon three findings: (1) the presence of increased aluminum in the cortex in AD (Crapper et al., 1973); (2) the experimental induction of NF in rabbits (Klatzo et al., 1965); (3) abnormal brain function in experimental aluminum toxicity, especially short-term memory (Crapper and Dalton, 1973). In cats poisoned with aluminum chloride ($AlCl_3$), functional abnormalities are described after cisternal injection, but apparently the most striking changes occur after direct hippocampal infusion of $AlCl_3$ (Crapper and Dalton, 1973a). In each case, a delay of about a week occurs after injection, so this affect is not considered to be due to the injection. At the same time (6–9 days) widespread NF are said to occur in the hippocampus and in large cells of the cortex. In this way, the evolution of aluminum-induced tangles is linked with behavioral changes. The EEG reveals no change in electrical activity in these animals at this time (Crapper and Dalton, 1973).

A hypothesis of neurotoxicity has evolved from these studies. Aluminum is taken up by neurons and soon afterward it can be detected in the nucleus bound to chromatin (De Coni et al., 1974). At some later time (6–9 days), NF occur in the cytoplasm of some of these cells due to increased or altered protein synthesis, presumably in response to the nuclear aluminum. The NF causes selective failure of neurotransmission by disrupting axon flow from the cell body to the distal neuron. This leads to altered behavior. Eventually, neuron death and cell loss occur. In other words, in susceptible neurons, aluminum induces abnormal protein synthesis as a primary effect

There are many contradictions in this concept both within the experimental model and in its application to AD. First, the distribution of the neuronal changes in the rabbit is quite unlike that of AD (Wisniewski et al., 1967). No changes are reported in the hippocampus, whereas brain stem and spinal cord are involved prominently. In the cat, Crapper and Dalton (1973a) state that the distribution of the lesions is similar to that observed by Wisniewski et al. (1967), yet they claim major involvement of the hippocampus, a distinct difference from Wisniewski et al. Early neuronal involvement is not described by Stercova (1966) and aluminum was not observed in neurons by Harris (1973).

Several investigators have reported inconsistent results in their studies of aluminum effects on protein synthesis. Only Exss and Summer (1973) report an abnormal basic proteon, but it is in neurites and not in the cell bodies. Neuronal RNA is said by Miller and Levine (1974) to be decreased, but Embree et al. (1967) found no change. All three authors agree that there is increased uptake of radioactive leucine by neuron cell bodies.

Apart from Crapper's study, the relationship between aluminum and human brain disease is far from clear. The epidemiology of aluminum encephalopathy consists of two cases. There is a single case of pulmonary fibrosis and encephalopathy (McGlaughlin et al., 1962) following heavy industrial exposure. Another patient is described as an alcoholic who had been diagnosed as having multiple sclerosis with no history of aluminum exposure (Lapresle et al., 1975). Pathologic examination of the patient with lead exposure has revealed 17 x normal aluminum, but otherwise the brain is normal with no evidence of Alzheimer's or Pick's disease. The other case has focal white-matter demyelination in which the aluminum is located, but no NF are present.

The metallic pathology of AD is also uncertain. Crapper et al. (1973) have only reported increased aluminum in homogenates of entire cortex. No one has reported increased metal in a neuronal enriched fraction. On the other hand, Duckett and Galle (1975) state that the aluminum is in SP and not in neurons. In their assay of isolated plaques, Austin et al. (1973) report a silicone content, but make no mention of increased aluminum. Finally, increased protein synthesis has not been reported in AD. These inconsistencies must be resolved before the aluminum hypothesis can be given credibility.

Slow Virus Infection

Concept of Slow Virus Infection

The idea of slow virus infection was originated by Sigurdsson (1954) following his studies of slowly progressive fatal diseases in Icelandic sheep. He believed that these disorders differed from usual infections in three ways: (1) an asymptomatic incubation period of months or years; (2) slow progression of clinical symptomatology, usually terminating in death; (3) selective species and organ involvement. The observation of a prolonged incubation period was of major importance, since it explained why transmission experiments had failed in earlier studies. It should be noted that Sigurdsson did not have a specific class of infectious agents in mind; in fact, he considered host factors as important as the character of the agent. In this sense, the term "slow virus infection" is a misnomer.

The accuracy of these concepts has been borne out by the recognition of diseases, particularly in the brain, as infectious in origin instead of degenerative disorders (Thormar, 1971). These conditions fall into two big categories: (1) those caused by conventional organisms (usually viral); (2) those related to unconventional agents, which have yet to be identified. For brain disease, the conventional organisms include measles, visna, lymphocytic choriomeningitis, and papova virus. They prominently involve the white matter and they seem to have no relevance for dementia (Fucillo et al., 1974). The major importance of these conventional agents is that, particularly in man, they are believed to exist only because a defective immune system permits their replication. This is very striking in subacute sclerosing panencephalitis where a massive amount of antibody is produced but is not effective in eliminating measles antigen (Thormar, 1971).

The nonconventional slow virus diseases include scrapie, transmissible mink encephalopathy (TME), kuru, and CJD. Common species susceptibilities have suggested that these may be due to the same etiologic agent, which has been attenuated by passage through different animals or which has a different host relationship. In each, the infectious agent is estimated to be smaller than a virus and to have responses to ionizing irradiation and UV light that are unlike those of conventional viruses. The scrapie agent is considered to be a prototype of this group and because of increased DNA synthesis in brains of scrapie-infected mice, the agent is conceived as being DNA in character. A single, instead of a double strand of DNA, plus a polysaccharide coat have been proposed as the basis for the differences from other DNA viruses (Adams, 1974).

All of these conditions are linked with long incubation periods up to 4 years in TME and CJD, 5 years in scrapie, and 20 years in kuru. During this time, the agent appears to be replicating within the lymphoreticular system. The scrapie agent can be detected in the spleen and lymph nodes of mice by the end of 1 month, but not in the brain until the fourth month (Eklund et al., 1967). The replication in the spleen and lymph nodes remains constant after 2 months, but does not elicit any pathologic change or immune response. The agent can only be detected by infectivity for other mice. The brain is the only organ that is altered by these agents. In contrast to other infected organs, the titer of scrapie in the brain continues to rise until death. Spongiform neuronopathy and gliosis are the characteristic changes in the brain (Lampert, 1972). The agent has not been identified, but it may be represented by aggregates of small electron-dense particles, which can be found in terminal axons and synapses of scrapie mice (Narang, 1974). These animals also have typical SP with thickened neurites and amyloid (Wisniewski et al., 1975). Transmission of the agent has been demonstrated by injection (kuru, scrapie, TME), by handling of infected brain (kuru), by tissue transplantation (CJD), and by contact (scrapie) (Asher et al., 1976).

Comparison of AD and Slow Virus Infection

The epidemiology of AD has implicated a genetic factor by an increased incidence among siblings and by hereditary disease. Species susceptibility is a characteristic of slow virus infection. Genotypic factors appear in kuru by female prevalence, in CJD by high incidence in Libyan Jews, and in scrapie by resistant sheep. All varieties of mink appear to be susceptible to TME, which enhances the contention that this is transmitted scrapie.

Geographic prevalence has been observed in all slow virus diseases involving unconventional agents. Scrapie in Scotland, TME in Wisconsin, kuru in New Guinea, and CJD in Libyan Jews all suggest that genotypic or contagious factors are involved in their transmission. Unfortunately, AD is found in all societies, so that regional occurence largely is not appreciated. However, if the surveys of rural Denmark and Sweden have credibility, the high incidence of AD is an indication that there is a greater incidence of senile dementia in these areas.

The clinical manifestations of AD suggest that there is primary involvement of the limbic system. In man, degeneration of the limbic system is recognized to occur with encephalitis, either of proven viral etiology in the case of herpes simplex or of suspected viral etiology as in the encephalitis associated with malignancy. Another characteristic of slow virus infections is the specificity of tissue damage with particular involvement of the brain. Even within the brain, a wide variety of regional change occurs, mainly subcortical in kuru and scrapie, but prominently cortical in TEM and CJD. In part, this appears to be species determined, since kuru becomes cortical in primates and scrapie becomes cortical in mink (Asher et al., 1976).

The effective disorders that occur prominently in the early stages of AD suggest that transmitter imbalance may be a basic problem. The recent finding of reduced cholinesterase (Bowen et al., 1976) enhances this contention greatly. An organic cause is offered by the progression to nonresponsiveness to psychoactive therapy, by the reduction of the dendritic network (Mehraein et al., 1975), and by the involvement of neurites and synapses in the SP.

There are not many conditions that are recognized to be destroyers of dendrites (Kreutzberg, 1975). The most widely studied abnormality of dendrites is that occurring in the cerebellum of the mutant mice, the weaver and staggerer, but these are considered to be developmental defects. Dendritic degeneration is also known to be caused by hyperbaric oxygen exposure at 5 atm or twice that which has been used as treatment of AD (Balentine, 1975). Pathogenicity of infectious agents for dendrites is reported by Lampert et al. (1975), who observed that dendritic involvement was a particular component in the spongiform changes of scrapie, kuru, and CJD. Blinzinger et al. (1975) have shown what they believe is flavovirus within dendrites, and Narang (1974) has shown possible scrapie agent in dendrites.

The SP is the most significant morphologic change found in AD. The thickened neurites and degenerating synapses have obvious importance for abnormal neurotransmission and the reduction of monoamine metabolites found in AD (Gottfried et al., 1969). A lack of specificity is indicated by their frequent occurrence in nondemented elderly brain, in Pick's disease, and in aging dog and monkey. It is worthy of note that Wisniewski and Terry (1973) have distinguished the plaques of Pick's disease and those in aged dogs and monkeys from AD because they lack abnormal fibrillar material. The amyloid plaques of kuru and CJD also differ from AD because they lack thickened neurites with abnormal neurofilaments. For this reason, a most notable observation was that the scrapie plaque was a complete plaque containing both amyloid and abnormal fibrils (Wisniewski et al., 1975). There is no other experimental model for complete plaque formation. Amyloid deposition has not been demonstrated among foci of thickned neurites induced by aluminum, even in studies up to 3 years (Crapper, 1976).

The presence of the amyloid reminds us that immunocompetence seems to be important, even if an autoimmune etiology is not credible. The predominant occurrence of AD between 75 and 89 years is necessarily linked with the decrease in immunocompetent units due to aging. A possible explanation of plaques in nondemented elderly is that they represent healed infection that is analogous to the Ghon complex of pulmonary tuberculosis. In this sense, immunologic collapse might be necessary for AD.

So the case for infectious etiology of AD seems very strong at this time. Some hereditary factor seems to be involved, but not in any kind of dominant role. Immunocompetence is probably critical and may be related to the hereditary factor. The infectious agent may be endogenous viral genetic material that has excaped immunosuppression, but more likely it is an exogenous agent relatively common in our environment. Vascular diesease and aging appear to have defaulted, acute confusion is just that, aluminum oxicity has to many contradictions, and autoimmune disease is attractive, but lacks actual support. The impact of this monograph hopefully will be a stimulation of the search for the infectious agent.

References

Adams, D.H. (1973). Nucleic acids as slow virus infections. Biochem. Soc. Trans. 1, 1061–1064

Adler, W.H. (1974): An autoimmune theory of aging. In: Theoretical Aspects of Aging. Rockstein, M. (ed.). New York: Academic Press, pp. 33–42

Agarwal, S.S., Blumberg, B.S., Gerstley, J.S., London, W.T., Sutnick, A.I., Loeb, L.A. (1970): DNA polymerase activity as an index of lymphocytic stimulation. Studies in Down's syndrome. J. Clin. Invest. 49, 161–169

Asher, D.M., Gibbs, C.J., Jr., Gajdusek, D.C. (1976): Pathogenesis of subacute spongiform encephalopathies. Ann. Clin. Lab. Sci. 6, 84–103

Austin, J.H., Rinehart, R., Williamson, T., Burcar, P., Russ, K., Nikaido, T., Lafrance, M. (1973): Studies in aging of the brain. III. Silicon levels in postmortem tissue and body fluids. Prog. Brain Res. 40, 486–495

Balentine, J.D. (1975): Dendritic degeneration following hyperbaric oxygen exposure. In: Physiology and Pathology of Dendrites. Kreutzberg, G.W. (ed.). New York: Raven Press. Adv. Neurol.12, 471–482

Ball, M.J. (1976): Neurofibrillary tangles and the pathogenesis of dementia. A quantitative study. Neuropathol. Appl. Neurobiol. 2, 395–410

Behan, P.O., Feldman, R.G. (1970): Serum proteins, amyloid and Alzheimer's disease. J. Am. Geriatr. Soc. 18, 792–797

Blessed, G., Tomlinson, B.E., Roth, M. (1968): The association between quantitative measures of dementia and of senile change in the cerebral grey matter of elderly subjects. Br. J. Psychiatry 114, 797–811

Blinzinger, K., Luh, S., Anzil, A.P. (1975): Virions and virus-associated structures within dendrites in an experimental flavovirus encephalomyelitis. In: Physiology and Pathology of Dendrites. Kreutzberg, G.W. (ed.). New York: Raven Press. Adv. Neurol. 12, 459–464

Bock, E., Kristensen, V., Refelson, O.J. (1974): Proteins in serum and cerebrospinal fluid in demented patients. Acta Neurol. Scand. 50, 91–102

Bowen, D.M., Smith, C.B., White, P., Davison, A.N. (1976): Neurotransmitter-related enzymes and indices of hypoxia in senile dementia and other abiotrophies. Brain 99, 459–496

Burch, P.R.J., Burwell, R.G. (1965): Self and not self. A clonal induction approach to immunology. Q. Rev. Biol. 40, 252–279

Burger, P.C., Vogel, F.S. (1973): The development of the pathologic changes of Alzheimer's disease and senile dementia in patients with Down's syndrome. Am. J. Pathol. 73, 457–468

Chisolm, J.J. (1970): Poisoning due to heavy metals. Pediatr. Clin. North Am. 17, 591–615

Cohen, A.S., Cathcart, E.S. (1974): Amyloidosis and immunoglobulins. Adv. Intern. Med. 19, 41–55

Crapper, D.R. (1976): Functional consequences of neurofibrillary degeneration. In: Neurobiology of Aging. Terry, R.D., Gershon, S. (eds.). New York: Raven Press, pp. 405–432

Crapper, D.R., Dalton, A.J. (1973): Aluminum induced neurofibrillary degeneration, brain electrical activity and alterations in acquisition and retention. Physiol. Behav. 10, 935–945

Crapper, D.R., Dalton, A.J. (1973a): Alterations in short-term retention, conditioned avoidance response acquisition and motivation following aluminum induced neurofribrollary degeneration. Phyiol. Behav. 10, 925–933

Crapper, D.R., Krishnan, S.S., Dalton, A.J. (1973): Brain aluminum distribution in Alzheimer's disease and experimental neurofibrillary degeneration. Science 180, 511–513

De Boni, U., Scott, J.W., Crapper, D.R. (1974): Intracellular aluminum binding: A histochemical study. Histochemistry 40, 31–37

Duckett, S., Galle, P. (1976): Mise en évidence de l'aluminum dans les plaques séniles de la maladie d'Alzheimer: Etude à la microsonde de Castaing. C.R. Acad. Sci. [D] (Paris) 282, 393–395

Dyggve, H., Clausen, J. (1970): The serum immunoglobulin level in Down's syndrome. Dev. Med. Child. Neurol. 12, 193–197

Eklund, C.M., Kennedy, R.C., Hadlow, W.J. (1967): Pathogenesis of scrapie virus infection in the mouse. J. Infect. Dis. 117, 15–22

Ellis, W.D., McCulloch, J.R., Corley, C.L. (1974): Presenile dementia in Down's syndrome. Neurology 24, 101–106

Embree, L.J., Hamberger, A., Sjöstrand, J. (1967): Quantitative cytochemical studies and histochemistry in experimental neurofibrillary degeneration. 26, 427–435

Exss, R.E., Summer, G.K. (1973): Basic proteins in neurons containing fibrillary deposits. Brain Res. 49, 151–164

Fucillo, D.A., Kurent, J.E., Sever, J.L. (1974): Slow virus diseases. Ann. Rev. Microbiol. 28, 231–264

Gottfries, C.G., Gottfries, I., Roos, B.E. (1969): Homovanillic acid and 5-hydroxyindoleacetic acid in the cerebrospinal fluid of patients with senile dementia, presenile dementia, and Parkinsonism. J. Neurochem. 16, 1341–1345

Greenfield, J.G. (1938): Discussion on the presenile dementias: Symptomatology, pathology, and differential diagnosis. Proc. R. Soc. Med. 31, 1450–1453

Gregory, L., Williams, R., Thompson, E. (1972): Leucocyte function in Down's syndrome and acute leukemia. Lancet 1, 1359–1361

Harris, A.B. (1973): Ultrastructure and histochemistry of alumina in cortex. Exp. Neurol. 38, 33–63

Hsia, D.Y., Justice, P., Smith, G.F., Dowhen, R.M. (1971): Down's syndrome. A critical review of the biochemical and immunological data. Am. J. Dis. Child. 121, 153–161

Kalter, S., Kelly, S. (1975): Alzheimer's disease. Evaluation of immunologic indices. N.Y. State J. Med. 75, 1222–1225

Klatzo, I., Wisniewski, H., Streicher, E. (1965): Experimental production of neurofibrillary degeneration. J. Neuropathol. Exp. Neurol. 24, 187–199

Kreutzberg, G.W. (1975): Physiology and Pathology of Dendrites. New York: Raven Press

Lampert, P.W., Gajdusek, D.C., Gibbs, C.J., Jr. (1975): Pathology of dendrites in subacute spongiform virus encephalopathies. In: Physiology and Pathology of Dendrites. Kreutzberg, G.W. (ed.). New York: Raven Press, pp. 465–470

Lampert, P.W., Gajdusek, D.C., Gibbs, C.J., Jr. (1972): Subacute spongiform virus encephalopathies. Am. J. Pathol. 68, 626–646

Lapresle, J., Duckett, S., Galle, P., Cartier, L. (1975): Documents cliniques, anatomiques et biophysiques dans une encéphalopathie avec présence de dépôts d'aluminium. C.R. Soc. Biol. (Paris) 169, 282–287

Larsson, T., Sjogren, T., Jacobson, G. (1963): Senile dementia. A clinical, sociomedical and genetic study. Acta Psychiatr. Scand. 39 (Suppl. 167), 1–227

McLaughlin, A.I.G., Kazanthis, G., King, E., Teare, D., Porter, R.J., Owen, R. (1962): Pulmonary fibrosis and encephalopathy associated with the inhalation of aluminium dust. Br. J. Ind. Med. 19, 253–263

McMenemey, W.H. (1968): Alois Alzheimer and his disease. In: Alzheimer's Disease and Related Disorders. Wolstenholme, G.E.W., O'Connor, M. (eds.). London: Churchill, pp. 5–9

Mehraein, P., Yamada, M., Tarnowska-Dziduszko, E. (1975): Quantitative study on dendrites and dendritic spines in Alzheimer's disease and senile dementia. In: Physiology and Pathology of Dendrites. Kreutzberg, G.W. (ed.). New York: Raven Press, Adv. Neurol. 12, 453–458

Miller, C.A., Levine, E.M. (1974): Effects of aluminum salts on cultured neuroblastoma cells. J. Neurochem. 22, 751–758

Nadler, H.L., Monteleone, P., Hsia, D.Y.Y. (1967): Enzyme studies during lymphocyte stimulation with phytohemagglutinin in Down's syndrome. Life Sci. 6, 2003–2008

Nandy, K. (1975): Significance of brain reactive antibodies in the serum of aged mice. J. Gerontol. 30, 412–416

Nandy, K. (1973): Brain-reactive antibodies in serum of aged mice. Prog. Brain Res. 40, 437–454

Nandy, K., Fritz, R.B., Threatt, J. (1975): Specificity of brain-reactive antibodies in serum of old mice. J. Gerontol. 30, 269–274

Narang, H.K. (1974): An electron microscopic study of the scrapie mouse and rat: Further observations on virus-like particles with ruthenium red and lanthanum nitrate as a possible trace and negative stain. Neurobiology 4, 349–363

Niklowitz, W.J., Mandybur, T.I. (1975): Neurofibrillary changes following childhood lead encephalopathy. J. Neuropathol. Exp. Neurol. 34, 445–455

Papez, J.W. (1937): A proposed mechanism of emotion. Arch. Neurol. Psychiatry 38, 725–743

Rundle, A.T., Clothier, B., Sudell, B. (1971): Serum IgD levels and infections in Down's syndrome. Clin. Chim. Acta 35, 389–393

Schlaepfer, W.W., Lynch, R.G. (1976): Immunofluorescent studies of neurofilaments in the peripheral and central nervous systems of rats and humans. (Abstr.) J. Neuropathol. Exp. Neurol. 35, 345

Shefer, V.F. (1972): Absolute number of neurons and thickness of the cerebral cortex during aging, senile and vascular dementia and Pick's and Alzheimer's diseases. Zhur. Neuropatol. Psikiat. Korsak. 72, 1024–1029

Sigurdson, B. (1954): Rida, a chronic encephalitis of sheep with general remarks on infections which develop slowly and some of their special characteristics. Br. Vet. J. 110, 341–354

Stercova, A. (1966): Dynamics of neurohistopathological changes in an epileptogenic focus produced by alumina cream in the rat. In: Comparative and Cellular Pathophysiology of Epilepsy. Servit, Z., Black, R. (eds.). New York: Excerpta Medica, pp. 247–255

Takeuchi, T., Morikawa, N., Matsumato, H., Shiraishi, H. (1962): A pathological study of minamata disease in Japan. Acta Neuropathol. 2, 40–57

Terry, R.D., Fitzgerald, C., Peck, A., Millern, J., Farmer, P. (1977): Cortical cell counts in senile dementia. J. Neuropathol. Exp. Neurol. 36, 633

Thormar, H. (1971): Slow infections of the central nervous system. Z. Neurol. 199, 1–23

Threatt, J., Nandy, K., Fritz, R. (1971): Brain-reactive antibodies in serum of old mice demonstrated by immunofluorescence. J. Gerontol. 26, 316–323

Tkach, J.R., Hokama, Y. (1970): Autoimmunity in chronic brain syndrome. A preliminary report. Arch. Gen. Psychiatry 23, 61–64

Victor, M. (1969): The amnesic syndrome and its anatomical basis. Can. Med. Assoc. J. 100, 1115–1125

Wisniewski, H.M., Bruce, M.E., Fraser, H. (1975): Infectious etiology of neuritic (senile) plaques in mice. Science 190, 1108–1110

Wisniewski, H.M., Terry, R.D. (1973): Re-examination of the pathogenesis of the senile plaque. In: Progress in Neuropathology. Zimmerman, H.M. (ed.). New York: Grune and Stratton, Vol. 2, pp. 1–25

Wisnieski, H.M., Narkiewicz, O., Wisniewska, K. (1967): Topography and dynamics of neurofibrillary degeneration in aluminum encephalopathy. Acta Neuropathol. 9, 127–133

Yakovlev, P.I. (1948): Motility, behavior and the brain. J. Nerv. Ment. Dis. 107, 313–335

Subject Index

Monographien aus dem Gesamtgebiete der Psychiatrie
Psychiatry Series

Herausgeber: H. Hippius,
W. Janzarik, M. Müller

1. Band: K. Hartmann
Theoretische und empirische Beiträge zur Verwahrlosungsforschung

Beiträge zur Verwahrlosungsforschung
2., neubearbeitete und erweiterte Auflage. 1977. 16 Abbildungen, 34 Tabellen. XII, 180 Seiten
ISBN 3-540-07925-4

2. Band: P. Matussek
Die Konzentrationslagerhaft und ihre Folgen
Mit R. Grigat, H. Haiböck,
G. Halbach, R. Kemmler,
D. Mantell, A. Triebel, M. Vardy,
G. Wedel
1971. 19 Abbildungen,
73 Tabellen. X, 272 Seiten
ISBN 3-540-05214-3

3. Band: A. E. Adams
Informationstheorie und Psychopathologie des Gedächtnisses
Methodische Beiträge zur experimentellen und klinischen Beurteilung mnestischer Leistungen
1971. 12 Abbildungen.
IX, 124 Seiten
ISBN 3-540-05215-1

4. Band: G. Nissen
Depressive Syndrome im Kindes- und Jugendalter
Beitrag zur Symptomatologie, Genese und Prognose
1971. 11 Abbildungen,
51 Tabellen. IX, 174 Seiten
ISBN 3-540-05493-6

5. Band: A. Moser
Die langfristige Entwicklung Oligophrener
Mit einem Vorwort von
Chr. Müller
1971. 4 Abbildungen,
30 Tabellen. X, 102 Seiten
ISBN 3-540-05599-1

6. Band: H. Feldmann
Hypochondrie
Leibbezogenheit. Risikoverhalten. Entwicklungsdynamik
1972. 36 Abbildungen,
5 Tabellen. VI, 118 Seiten
ISBN 3-540-05753-6

7. Band: S. Meyer-Osterkamp,
R. Cohen
Zur Größenkonstanz bei Schizophrenen
Eine experimentalpsychologische Untersuchung. Mit einem einführenden Geleitwort von
H. Heimann
1973. 5 Abbildungen.
VII, 91 Seiten
ISBN 3-540-06147-9

8. Band: K. Diebold
Die erblichen myoklonisch-epileptisch-dementiellen Kernsyndrome
Progressive Myoklonusepilepsien – Dyssinergia cerebellaris myoclonica – myoklonische Varianten der drei nachinfantilen Formen der amaurotischen Idiotie
1973. 31 Abbildungen.
IX, 254 Seiten
ISBN 3-540-06117-7

9. Band: C. Eggers
Verlaufsweisen kindlicher und präpuberaler Schizophrenien
1973. 3 Abbildungen.
IX, 250 Seiten
ISBN 3-540-06163-0

10. Band: M. Schrenk
Über den Umgang mit Geisteskranken
Die Entwicklung der psychiatrischen Therapie vom „moralischen Regime" in England und Frankreich zu den „psychischen Curmethoden" in Deutschland
1973. 20 Abbildungen.
IX, 194 Seiten
ISBN 3-540-06267-X

11. Band: Heinz Schepank
Erb- und Umweltfaktoren bei Neurosen
Tiefenpsychologische Untersuchungen an 50 Zwillingspaaren
Unter Mitarbeit von P. E. Becker,
A. Heigl-Evers, C. O. Köhler,
Helga Schepank, G. Wagner
1974. 1 Abbildung, 82 Tabellen.
VIII, 227 Seiten
ISBN 3-540-06647-0

12. Band: L. Ciompi, C. Müller
Lebensweg und Alter der Schizophrenen
Eine katamnestische Langzeitstudie bis ins Senium
27 Fallbeispiele.

1976. 23 Abbildungen,
48 Tabellen. IX, 242 Seiten
ISBN 3-540-07567-4

13. Band: L. Süllwold
Symptome schizophrener Erkrankungen
Uncharakteristische Basisstörungen
1977. 15 Tabellen.
VIII, 112 Seiten
ISBN 3-540-08203-4

14. Band: **The Apallic Syndrome**
Editors: G. Dalle Ore,
F. Gerstenbrand, C. H. Lücking,
G. Peters, U. H. Peters
With the editorial assistance of
E. Rothemund
1977. 67 figures, 17 tables.
XV, 259 pages
ISBN 3-540-08301-4

15. Band: O. Benkert
Sexuelle Impotenz
Neuroendokrinologische und pharmakotherapeutische Untersuchungen
1977. 33 Abbildungen,
20 Tabellen. VIII, 139 Seiten
ISBN 3-540-08427-4

16. Band: R. Avenarius
Der Größenwahn
Erscheinungsbilder und Entstehungsweise
1978. VI, 98 Seiten
ISBN 3-540-08547-5

17. Band: **Psychiatrische Epidemiologie**
Geschichte, Einführung und ausgewählte Forschungsergebnisse
Herausgeber: H. Häfner
1978. 20 Abbildungen,
91 Tabellen, XII, 252 Seiten
ISBN 3-540-08629-3

18. Band: **Transmethylations and the Central Nervous System**
Edited by V. M. Andreoli,
A. Agnoli, C. Fazio
1978. 45 figures, 42 tables.
Approx. 190 pages
ISBN 3-540-08693-5

19. Band: **Psychiatrische Therapie-Forschung**
Ethische und juristische Probleme
Herausgeber: H. Helmchen,
B. Müller-Oerlinghausen
1978. XII, 180 Seiten
ISBN 3-540-08732-X

Springer-Verlag
Berlin Heidelberg New York

H. Prinzhorn

Artistry of the Mentally Ill

A Contribution to the Psychology and Psychopathology of Configuration

Translation from the Second German Edition: E. von Brockdorff. With an Introduction by J.L. Foy 1972. 187 figures (16 in color). XXIII, 274 pages ISBN 3-540-05508-8

From the reviews of the German edition: "When first published in 1922, this book was almost the first attempt to analyse art works of psychotics. This new edition shows that the work is still very important as a reference book and outstanding in the study of art by mental patients. The reproduced material is exceptional and includes many colour reproductions. The book also offers a survey of the relevant literature until the time in question. ... The new psychoanalytical approach, exploring the unconscious, has given new understanding to the meaning of any artistic production. This could be applied to the production of perfectly normal artists as well as to that of psychotics..."

The British Journal of Psychiatry

"In this beautifully printed volume are many black and white and colored illustrations used by the author to clarify his discussion of the role of expressive artistic production in the understanding of various psychiatric disturbances. The reprinting of this classical work by Prinzhorn may permit some of his ideas to infiltrate the thinking of a large number of students and clinicians."

Psychological Reports (USA)

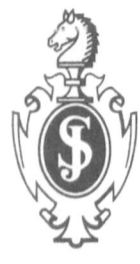

Springer-Verlag
Berlin
Heidelberg
New York